Roy Masters was a first-grade rugby league coach for ten years and was named coach of the year three times, and Western Suburbs coach of the century. He was an inaugural member of the Australian Sports Commission and served for 23 years. Masters has been a senior writer with the *Sydney Morning Herald* for over 20 years.

HIGHER RICHER SLEAZIER

How drugs and money are changing sport forever

ROY MASTERS

ALLEN&UNWIN

First published by Allen & Unwin in 2010

Allen & Unwin
83 Alexander Street
Crows Nest NSW 2065
Australia
Phone: (61 2) 8425 0100
Fax: (61 2) 9906 2218
Email: info@allenandunwin.com
Web: www.allenandunwin.com

Cataloguing-in-Publication details are available
from the National Library of Australia
www.librariesaustralia.nla.gov

ISBN: 978 1 74175 917 4 (pbk.)

Typeset in Australia by Midland Typesetters in 12/15 pt Warnock Pro

10 9 8 7 6 5 4 3 2 1

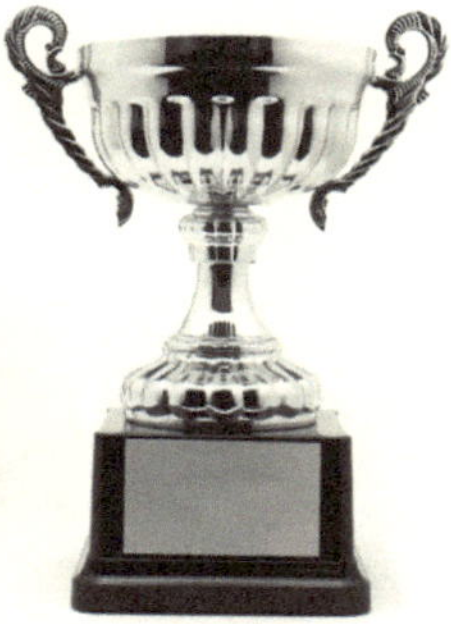

CONTENTS

To my mother Olga, a great Australian writer who gave me a love of words.

ONE 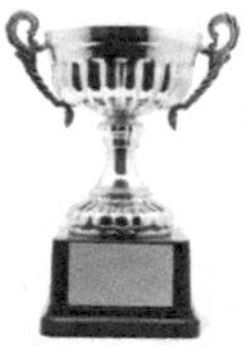 LET THE GAMES BEGIN

Fans complain sport is now merely a business, but the opposite applies and is even more unnerving: business is often a sport. Pluck the ostentatious braces of many company directors and a sporting metaphor falls out. An executive search team, justifying its recruitment of bankers who contributed to the global financial crisis, said, 'Someone who fumbles on the last play is likely to hold the ball tightly next time'.

When the Australian Government announced changes to superannuation in the wake of the crisis, the headline read, 'Moving the Goal Posts'. Inflation has even taken hold of the effort of footballers, with last week's 'We're going to give it 110%', superseded by this week's '120%'. *The Sydney Morning Herald*, the newspaper where I have worked for over twenty years, now combines business and sport in a single section.

The multimillionaires who sit on the boards of football clubs have become indistinguishable from the athletes they pay, certainly in terms of their big salaries, expensive toys, win-at-all-costs mentality and the heady celebrity mix with film stars. Rugby league, once described by jailed media baron Lord Conrad Black as 'that arcane sport', attracts Oscar winner Russell Crowe as an owner of South Sydney and supermodel Sarah Murdoch as one of Manly's 'Eagle Angels' booster group. Sarah's media magnate husband Lachlan Murdoch, the son of News Corporation boss Rupert, is the reason News Limited will not sell its 67 per cent shareholding in the Brisbane Broncos. Lachlan is the NRL club's No. 1 fan and once sat in the coach's box.

With the mega-salaries paid these days to those endowed with prodigious physical talents, sport has become the new establishment, and the old establishment—business tycoons, politicians and even the nobility—have obtruded on sport in search of respectability. The International Olympic Committee is laced with royals, including Princess Anne, the only female athlete at the Montreal Olympics of 1976 (on Great Britain's equestrian team) not required to undertake a sex test. Business/celebrity/nobility castes have effectively switched positions with the sports stars. Players at NRL clubs wear pinstriped suits to games and drink water afterwards, while their directors, such as car-czar Nick Politis, chairman of the Sydney Roosters, watch on in upmarket sneakers and expensive casual clothes and quaff beer and wine in their private suite.

Sir Allen Stanford, an American financier with Antiguan citizenship, strutted like the bullfighter in *Carmen* during a Twenty20 match between England and the Stanford Superstars, a West Indies-based team. He barged in and out of the dressings rooms at Antigua's Stanford Cricket Ground and flirted shamelessly with the wives and girlfriends of the English players, bouncing one, who was pregnant, on his knee. The players, competing for US$1 million each in prize money in this winner-takes-all match, were mortified, but played on. To announce the Stanford Super Series, Sir Allen had earlier landed his helicopter on Lord's sacred turf, while officials of the England and Wales

Cricket Board obsequiously lined the impromptu landing pad, posing with him beside a crate containing US$20 million in cash. The Stanford Superstars won the Antigua match, with England captain Kevin Pietersen telling his counterpart, Chris Gayle, afterwards, 'You needed the money more than us'.

Less than a year later, Stanford was charged with a US$8 billion fraud and many sportsmen, including cricketers and golfers, were his victims.

Australia's Formula 1 driver Mark Webber attends a cocktail party, picks carefully from passing plates of fat-free food, before going home to his wife—his former corporate advisor—on the outskirts of London. Meanwhile, his fellow drivers joke about the sexual activities of diminutive grand prix despot Bernie Ecclestone and his soon-to-be-divorced, very tall wife, quipping, 'I wonder who puts him up to it'. Playboy Italian Flavio Briatore is a friend and co-owner with Ecclestone of soccer club Queens Park Rangers. Briatore considers himself coach of QPR, sending the selected team back to the manager if he does not agree with the lineup. For a time, he was managing director of the Renault Formula 1 team, boasting to English newspapers, 'Bernie and I speak on the phone five times a day'.

While this suggests sport is the glue of the rich, it also reflects the many conflicts of interest which pervade the sport–business relationship. (Such men usually contemptuously dismiss these conflicts as of interest only to pesky journalists. When I raised with Australian Rugby Union boss John O'Neill his then conflict as chair of Events NSW, meaning his responsibility of allocating Wallaby games around the nation collided with his obligation to deliver them to New South Wales, O'Neill had a novel answer. He quoted the late billionaire Kerry Packer who once growled, 'If you haven't got a conflict, you haven't got an interest.') As it transpired, the close relationship between Ecclestone, the man charged with running Formula 1, and Briatore, the boss of one of the teams, was challenged when Briatore was sacked by Renault for his involvement in a race-fixing scam. But Briatore also owns holiday resorts in Italy and Kenya, plus The Billionaire nightclub in Sardinia and the Billionaire Italian Couture fashion label. He has been romantically linked with supermodels and had a child with one. He is horizontally integrated via his companies and contacts to provide girls, grog and gifts for his past drivers and present soccer players. But who is having the fun?

Whereas the late George Best, one of soccer's best ever players, once quipped he had lost almost all his earnings on wine, women and song ('The rest I wasted', he declared), now it's the owners who are partying. It's all very symmetrical, to say nothing of lucrative for businessmen and athletes—whether you're talking about executives for whom money has become just another way of keeping score, or about sports stars for whom scoring now means making money, as opposed to buying drugs or bedding girls.

And do the business owners of sport really care about their star performers when they describe them as 'assets'? When US baseball's highest paid player, the New York Yankees' Alex Rodriguez, confessed to a long-suspected history of taking performance-enhancing drugs, he was one year into a ten-year deal. The Yankees obviously wrestled with the economics of paying out 'A-Rod's' contract and receiving little compensation. General Manager Brian Cashman said at a press conference, 'We have nine years of Alex remaining and we want it to be nine terrific years. He is a huge investment. This is an asset that's currently in crisis and we will do everything we can to protect this asset and move forward with this asset.' That's three mentions of the word asset in one sentence. When Rodriguez was originally 'traded' to the Yankees, he was a 'blue chip recruit' but presumably now he is a 'fixed asset'. The asset paid off late in 2009 when the Yankees won the World Series, New York's first since 2000. Not surprisingly, the American media lists the pre, post and current season movements of players under the headings 'trades'.

I have been a participant and observer of sport for many years—coaching first-class professional sport and then covering it in the media for 25 years, including attending several Olympic Games. Spanning my coaching/media careers there was a 23-year period when I was an inaugural board member of the Australian Sports Commission, the federal government body responsible for funding sport. These roles placed me in a unique position to view sport from a number of angles. What follows is my observation of the use of drugs by sportspeople (Chapter Two), the globalisation of sport (Chapter Three) and game fixing, tanking and the tactics of intimidation (Chapter Four)—in short, how drugs and money are changing sport forever. In Chapter Five, entitled 'Further', I look at the rise of the black athlete and the problems facing women's sport and their futures. The position of the modern athlete as role model and the growing divide between fan and sporting hero is covered in Chapter Six, adding fame to the list of what influences the direction of sport today. A thread through all of the chapters is what I see as the failure of the administrators of professional and amateur sports to truly care for their charges, despite many of them having once been former sports champions themselves.

The G7 conference of nations addressed the relationship between sport and business in 1989, setting up a study group in the Financial Action Task Force that combats money laundering among other duties. It took two decades to produce its 'Money Laundering through the Football Sector' report, which noted that the big money flowing into sport brought higher risk of fraud and corruption. 'Sport can also be used as a channel to launder dirty money', the report said. It identified the rugby codes, soccer, cricket, horse and car racing as the sports most vulnerable: 'There are connections between criminal organisations (including international organised crime) and the world of football . . . Social prestige is an important factor . . . Popular sport can be a route for criminals to become celebrities by associating with famous people and moving upwards to powerful circles within established society.'

In Melbourne, where the AFL takes on the status of a secular religion, the links between footballers and criminals became evident during the notorious gang wars. The AFL's best player during the 1990s, Wayne Carey, was a character witness for one of the city's most notorious gangsters, Jason Moran. Moran was gunned down while sitting in his car with an associate watching his kids play Auskick, the modified rules version of AFL. Four years later, a Collingwood player, Alan Didak, won over by a few free drinks in a nightclub paid for by a member of a feared motorcycle gang, accompanied the bikie on a high-speed journey through the city's streets, with the bikie shooting at a police station. That bikie was later arrested, found guilty and sent to jail for murdering a young father and seriously wounding a backpacker, both of whom objected to him dragging a woman from a nightclub while other pedestrians were hurrying one morning to work. A West Coast Eagles player celebrated a win in front of TV cameras by joining his wrists together, as if handcuffed, sending a message of fealty to a recently jailed member of a Perth motorcycle gang.

The G7 report pointed out the criminal connection can begin at the grassroots level of the game, explaining that amateur sports were vulnerable to infiltration by criminals because the often inexperienced, under-skilled volunteers who ran the clubs were prone to hide embarrassments for fear of losing sponsors. This made them vulnerable to monetary gifts from criminals, satisfying both the club that needed the money and the donor who welcomed the patron status. 'The criminal is buying an entrance ticket to a social milieu', the report said. As the criminal progresses deeper into the social milieu, he can gather information from players that becomes extremely lucrative because of the vast network of gambling outlets available.

Australia is vulnerable to exploitation by an Asian crime syndicate with an established reach into Europe, according to one of the world's leading investigative journalists, Canada's Declan Hill. 'The people who are doing this have targeted your country and will be destroying your sports within three to five years', Hill told the annual conference of the Australian and New Zealand Sports Law Association in September 2009. 'You have a brief window of opportunity to stop them coming in or they will wreak havoc here.' Hill, who spent four years reseaching his book *The Fix*, said the illegal sports gambling racket in Asia dwarfed legitimate agencies. He claimed it killed off the Chinese premier league because corruption was so bad, teams walked from the pitch mid match.

Australia's exposure to gambling, Hill claimed, is related to our shared time zone with Asia, our obsession with sport and gambling, and the proliferation of elite national competitions, some involving athletes who were not highly paid. 'They play in these high profile games but if [fixers] were to come to a certain team with $10,000, it's probably more than many of their junior players see in a week,' he said, possibly unaware some A-League soccer players and netballers would not receive $10,000 in a month.

A month after Hill's warning, the world governing body of soccer, FIFA, called an emergency executive meeting in Capetown to confront revelations of match fixing across at least nine European leagues involving up to 200 matches. German-based betting syndicates were suspected of bribing players, coaches, referees and officials to fix games for Asian betting syndicates for alleged profits of more than $16 million. With Australia now belonging to the Asian Football Confederation and expanding its A-League from eight teams to twelve, partly to access the rich Asian club tournament, questions were asked whether the A-League could become a target for match fixers. Ironically, the first ex-player to spring to Australia's defence against these suggestions was a convicted match fixer. Former Socceroo striker Abbas Saad, fined for match fixing while playing in Singapore for the Malaysia league, said, 'To be honest, I don't think these blokes would be interested in Australia. The market is too small.' Saad, now a TV commentator in Singapore, explained, 'The gamblers are looking for the big markets, which is why they look to Europe. The only thing that could be an issue is that Australia is now part of Asia, so the AFC games might be a target. Who's to say?'

Australia's major sports bosses have certainly embraced the gambling dollar. Hill's warning came as the AFL, the nation's biggest winter sport, moved towards live coverage of matches, meaning gamblers could punt online or by mobile phone in real time. Some of these exotic bets may eventually include whether a player misses his next attempt at goal. The AFL, like the NRL, is sponsored by a corporate bookmaker and betting exchange, Betfair, which accepts bets on a team losing a match. Yet, while the big sports accept these sponsorships, they do nothing to stop clubs naming wrong lineups that deceive the punter. Sure, the masquerade team is designed to confuse the opposition, but the smokescreen also causes punters to make wrong decisions. Even where token amounts of money are involved, such as with office-tipping competitions, this deceit undermines interest in the game. There are significant bragging rights attached to winning a tipping competition and the weekend results are usually the main topic of conversation at the Monday morning coffee break. Yet the AFL and NRL do little to stop champion players being named in teams and withdrawn an hour before kick off. Some clubs injury lists have more misdirections than you would witness in a David Copperfield show.

It's over 30 years since Chicago Cubs baseball owner Philip K. Wrigley complained baseball was too much of a sport to be a business and too much of a business to be a sport. The collision between sport and business was brutally demonstrated in Australia's biggest sports story of the new millennium: the 2010 train wreck of the NRL club, the Melbourne Storm. The News Limited-owned club was cruelly punished by the half News Limited-owned NRL for salary cap breaches. The interest of the footballers (sport) were subjugated to the interest of News Limited (business) as Rupert Murdoch's media company ran an agenda to protect their commercial interests and corporate reputation.

The club admitted to overspending $1.7 million during the previous five years and was punished with the loss of five premierships (two major and three minor), fined $1.6 million and forced to play the 2010 season for zero premiership points. In so far as the NRL salary cap average slightly less than

$4 million during this period, the excess payments to players represented a 10 per cent budget blowout. Yet sportswriters, who regularly fudge their weekly expenses, and media executives, who use corporate credit cards for expensive lunches, savaged the Storm.

News Limited was entitled to be angry the club officials had deceived the corporation by diverting marketing income into players' pockets, forcing up the annual $6 million subsidy the media organisation paid the club that operates in a non-rugby league market. Senior News Limited executives did not deny their horrendous conflict of interest, cleverly described by one writer as a situation where the hand that feeds and the mouth that bites belong to the same being. But the media company's senior executives, who should have exercised a closer watch on the spending in Melbourne, were in frequent dialogue with the NRL chief executive, David Gallop, in the days leading up to the announcement of the horrendous penalties. Some insiders even profited from the knowledge of the impending penalties with a series of bets placed on the Storm to win the wooden spoon. Bookmakers suspended betting on the Storm coming last, tipping journalists of the coming saga and igniting the firestorm of publicity.

The inescapable conclusion was News Limited wanted heavy sanctions to retrieve their reputation, trashed by their lack of supervision and undermined by their conflict of interest. They wanted a penalty that showed no favouritism to their 100 per cent-owned club. The saga was all very reminiscent of the Salt Lake City bribery scandal where the US city won the right to host the 2002 Winter Olympics by bribing IOC officials. Then-IOC president Juan Antonio Samaranch and his executive board protested that they had no knowledge of the entrenched vote buying in the Olympic movement. News Limited, like Samaranch, stood accused of being complicit or incompetent.

Storm players, who had transferred to the club on modest contracts to benefit from the superior coaching at the Storm, had their premiership cancelled, their personal histories marked with an asterisk and their motivation to win scuttled. The NRL should never have taken the premierships away, particularly the 2007 flag, which was won with an acknowledged $200,000 overspend, slightly more than the Roosters had admitted to after winning the 2002 title. There was also an alternative to the decision to stop the Storm accruing points in 2010: it could have ruled the Storm start the subsequent season on minus premiership points, in the same way AFL and NFL clubs are punished for salary cap breaches by denying them top-draft choices in successive years.

The four independent directors of the Storm took out a writ in the Victorian Supreme Court to overturn the penalties, while the two News Limited employed directors stood aside from the decision. Other NRL clubs waited nervously for exposures of their own breaches. The NRL salary cap had been pitched at a level equal to the capacity to the pay of the poorest club, meaning those with more money to spend had to find devious ways to survive in a world that had changed irrevocably from the big salaries of Super League and the advent of professionalism in rugby union. Now, all of sport is at the crossroads. Some of our major sporting organisations are perceived by their once-adoring public to be exclusively a business—with salary caps, drafts, next-generation broadcasting rights and 'creature comforts'—while many of the once-amateur Olympic disciplines, administered from the kitchen table of a well-meaning volunteer, are seen as too much of a sport to be a business. A letter writer to the Melbourne *Age* newspaper, following the explosive January 2008 second cricket Test between Australia and India at the Sydney Cricket Ground, best summed up the confusion and anger fans felt over the commercially driven, win-at-all-costs, hypocritical behaviour of the Australian players: 'Now that the "sport" has been completely removed from cricket, perhaps the results can be listed in the business section, and reports on individual cricketers in the personal finance pages.' (9 January 2008). We can imagine the letter writer asking, What has happened to the game's poetry? 'There's no money in poetry', answered the English poet Robert Graves, adding, 'But there is no poetry in money, either'.

India's captain Anil Kumble was so incensed at the behaviour of the Australian players he echoed the words used by Australia's captain Bill Woodfull describing England's tactics during the infamous Bodyline series of 1932–33. 'I think only one side was playing in the spirit of the game', Kumble said, prompting one clever sub-editor to dub the Sydney Test, 'Bollyline', a reference to India's film-star industry which has invested heavily in Indian cricket.

If Australian players were too professional in their approach to victory, the administrators behaved like beseiged amateurs, surrendering shamefully to the mighty rupee, as they bowed to India's threats to take their bat and ball and go home. India's politicians had already achieved what the Indian players could not do on the field. An appeal against spinner Harbhajan's Singh's suspension for racial abuse of Australian all-rounder Andrew Symonds was lodged by an official who was also a minister in the Indian Government. The ICC (International Cricket Council) quickly allowed it, meaning Harbhajan could play until it was heard . . . conveniently after the final Test match in Adelaide.

Then, with threats of an India-bound jet warming its motors on the Adelaide tarmac and the remaining one-day matches of the tour possibly being abandoned, India succeeded in having the charge against the spinner downgraded to one of abusive language—to which he pleaded guilty.

India, the world's second largest nation, supplies 70 per cent of global cricket's revenue, sustaining the Dubai-based ICC. Its cricket board has been described as a mixture of 'hypercapitalism and feudalism'; because many of its board members are politicians, they react to their constituents' wishes rather than the interests of the game. When voters are burning effigies of match referees or umpires on the streets of Mumbai, the Board of Control for Cricket in India looks ahead to the next election more than the next ICC meeting. It will be fascinating to observe how the next ICC chairman—former Australian Prime Minister John Howard— rules the sport . . . and India.

The norms and traditions in every cricket-playing nation, including the old powers, England and Australia, will be challenged as Indian cricket exercises the control that derives from its massive wealth. This was demonstrated in the return series in India later in 2008, when India threatened to play an opening batsman who had been banned for one Test for elbowing Australia's Shane Watson. As early as November 2001, the Indian team had threatened to boycott an up-coming series against England because they were angry with the decisions of match referee Mike Denness during a tour of South Africa. Denness had had the temerity to level charges against some players, including for excessive appealing—one of India's problems with Australia in Sydney.

Even cricket's nineteenth-century colossus, the legendary English captain, Dr W.G. Grace, abided by the umpire's rulings. He once reputedly picked up a dislodged bail and replaced it on the stumps after he was bowled, saying to the umpire, 'Windy day, isn't it?' The umpire directed him to the pavilion. But during 'Bollyline', India challenged the umpire, threatening the one universal principle that has always held international sport together: the role of the umpire as impartial arbiter is inviolable. An Indian official telephoned ICC chief executive Malcolm Speed asking him not to appoint to the Perth Test umpire Steve Bucknor, who had been the centre of the Second Test controversy. Speed consulted with the Australian team and, seeking to defuse the situation, dropped Bucknor. The ICC then expected the public to believe the West Indian umpire was not replaced, declaring in its press release that it wasn't 'due to any representations made by any team or individual'.

Bucknor had given evidence to the Sydney match referee on the dispute between Harbhajan and Symonds, but was out of the country by the time of the appeal. Justice John Hansen, a New Zealand judge, heard the appeal, dismissing the charge against the Indian for racial abuse and downgrading it to merely verbal abuse. Hansen later addressed a sport law forum held in Melbourne and observed: 'Umpire Bucknor, who was closer to the action than most, but who was unavailable by the time of the hearing in front of me, simply described the exchange to the match referee as the usual sort of "argy bargy" that one gets on the field. So what one umpire thought was usual "argy bargy" in fact led to a furore that threatened the suspension of one of the most important cricket tours of modern times, again highlighting the confusion that we are confronted with.' You get the feeling umpire Bucknor, like the

Indian players, thought the exchange was all part of sport, while the Indian administrators knew they were in a business.

Judge Hansen was highly critical of Symonds, who admitted in the hearing he objected to Harbhajan patting Australian bowler Brett Lee on the bum after Lee bowled an excellent yorker to him. 'My objection was that a Test match is no place to be friendly with opposition players', Symonds told the hearing. Judge Hansen wrote in his judgement, 'If that is his view, I hope it is not one shared by all international cricketers. It would be a sad day for cricket if it is.' Similar sentiments were expressed by one of Hansen's fellow judges, Justice J.A. Tadgell in Victoria's Court of Appeal. After hearing the appeal by AFL footballer, Greg Williams against a suspension, Tadgell said of the hours spent in the courtroom and the trees felled to read the evidence: 'There are those who would regard football also as a sport, but I don't recall in the course of this appeal reading the word "sport" or hearing it mentioned by counsel.'

While it may conform to popular opinion to accuse Australian cricketers, footballers and Indian officials and AFL club bosses of being too business oriented, it is equally possible to charge some of the non-professional sports with not being sufficiently so minded. Having witnessed the muddled thinking of some team managers at ten Olympic Games and five Commonwealth Games, I find it hard to escape the notion that the only amateurs left in both movements are the officials. One of the hardest tasks in modern sport is to convince a long-serving official of the once-amateur games to surrender his blazer.

Amateur boxing, the last of the lilywhites in the sense their athletes, along with equestrians, are the only competitors not allowed to be paid—an example, both in Australia and at the international level, of a sport devoid of business acumen. As a board member of the Australian Sports Commission I witnessed many volatile exchanges between the directors of Boxing Australia and the long-term ruler of the sport, Arthur Tunstall.

At a BA board meeting in Surfers Paradise held in April 2000, Tunstall was accused of triple dipping—he had claimed airfares to the World Championships in Houston, Texas, from the Australian Olympic Committee, Boxing Australia and the AIBA (the International Association). The then 81-year-old Arthur was told that his creative accounting would be forgiven provided he didn't stand for office at the next BA elections. A penitent Arthur agreed, but the lure of power proved too great. At the next AGM, he threw US$1090 on the table as a peace offering. It was money he admitted to claiming twice for his business-class travel to Houston, but insisted he had kept it in a drawer for a year, always intending to re-pay it. Arthur then put his name forward for re-election on the nomination of Michael Hodgman QC, the former Tasmanian federal parliamentarian nicknamed 'the Mouth from the South'. Arthur lost 5–4 with two abstaining.

When delegates sought more information from Tunstall on other travel, including a trip to an AIBA conference in Turkey, the minutes record him saying, 'I am not going to say anything. I should never have put the bloody money on the table today.' The BA secretary later went to a bank to verify the American currency was old notes, as Arthur had claimed, rather than monies recently exchanged. A bank teller assured the secretary the money was aged. During the meeting, which was taped, Hodgman succeeded in having withdrawn a motion that would have effectively disqualified Tunstall for life from holding a position with BA, or from representing it in any way, and would have erased his name from a perpetual trophy. Hodgman then challenged the president of BA, Sol Spitalnic, to the top office but failed 8–3 and walked from the room and the sport.

Tunstall wears his advancing age as if it were a bathrobe and slippers, not caring how he looks to his critics in the media or government. Yet there was a hint of sadness that a web of recrimination and rancour had replaced his network of friends. When I asked Arthur after the meeting if he believed the board feared him, he said, 'Correct. I'm fucked if I can understand what they are frightened about.' Power.

The bridge between Tunstall and his old friend, Spitalnic, was still trembling from yet an earlier feud when Tunstall had lost his last significant Commonwealth Games post, being voted off as Oceania delegate and sacked as national secretary of amateur boxing after 47 years of service. Yet, despite all the political manoeuvring against him, he told me he would never challenge Spitalnic for the presidency of BA. It seems an ancient bond—the Masonic Order—was more important. Tunstall said, 'Sol and I had a shake of the hand of a certain organisation on that.'

Spitalnic subsequently walked away from amateur boxing to care for his ill wife, leaving Tunstall to run New South Wales as his own personal feifdom. It took another eight years before the new hierarchy of BA could oust Arthur. In November 2009, BA's council voted 10–2 to disband the association of Australia's biggest state on the recommendation of a judiciary review of complaints, including allegations of racism against Tunstall. One submission claimed he opposed sending an Aboriginal boxer to the Olympics because, 'We need people who know how to use a knife and a fork.' On the day his incredible 60-year reign came to an end, Tunstall said, 'The real story is BA couldn't handle me telling it straight. They've wanted me out for ages and now they've finally succeeded.'

The 2008 SCG cricket test against India was a salutary reminder on why sport is so important to Australians. It had everything—the obsesssion with winning overtaking respect for the opposition; the interests of the team opposed to the morality of the individual; gamesmanship versus sportsmanship; technology versus human error; cultural clashes; bad luck and good fortune; honesty and hypocrisy. Prominent Australians—from the governor-general to Hall of Famers, such as athletes Herb Elliott and Rob de Castella and yachtsman John Bertrand—made public speeches and issued press releases. It dominated newspaper reports and TV and radio headline news for a fortnight after Australia's improbable win at the end of the second last over on the final day. It demonstrated the beauty and ugliness of cricket: a game of slow grace and deathly quick changes of fortune. What other game on earth is played over five days, yet can be decided in the disappearing minutes?

Players refused to walk, standing their ground when it seemed everyone at the SCG heard a snick; catches were claimed when TV replays indicated the ball first touched the ground; Ricky Ponting, the Australian captain, should have been given out when he deflected a ball and yet he survived, only to be wrongly given out leg before wicket when a ball deflected off his bat onto his pads. It was an easy mistake for the umpire to make, with the bat so close to the pad as to make the deflection almost imperceptible, but Ponting glared at the ageing Bucknor and stood his ground momentarily before hurling his bat through the door when he finally entered the dressing room. Ponting reported Indian spinner Harbhajan for calling Australia's only black player, Symonds, a 'monkey', while the Indians accused wrist spinner Brad Hogg of calling two of them 'bastards'. Suddenly, the professional, business-oriented game of cricket had descended to a schoolboy game of cowboys and Indians, spiced by name calling. How could professional men paid so handsomely behave so poorly? Isn't this sort of behaviour more associated with sub-district cricket and pub footy?

The reality is that players in amateur sports tend to behave better. An ideal game is played without referees or umpires, and in many village green cricket matches the batting team act as umpires. Sure, everyone appeals and no-one walks but when a batsman stands his ground and the umpire asks him directly whether he snicked the ball, it's one thing to stay and another thing entirely to lie to a team mate. The word amateur derives from Latin *amator* ('lover') and in that sense these are true amateurs. They are also amateurs in the currently outmoded but nonethelesss admirable sense that their effort is their own reward and they don't want it sullied by cheating and lies.

Can there be a better example of sport played for its own sake than the games of soccer between English and German troops on Boxing Day 1914? A Christmas truce had been informally called the day before and, after beer, plum pudding and photos of loved ones had been exchanged by the soldiers on either side, they did what most young men do . . . played a game of scratch football. As news of the truce spread down the line, games involved up to 100 men, with tins used for balls, helmets and bayonets for goal posts and the field a crater-filled quagmire. But, true to a recurring theme of this book, the administrators—in this case the top brass—stuffed it up. The high command on both sides feared the fraternising ran the risk of humanising the enemy and the truce lasted a day. Liverpool manager, Bill Shankly, famously said when asked whether football was a matter of life or death, 'No, it's more important than that'. The Boxing Day 1914 game wasn't what Shankly had in mind but it was an occasion when sport was more important than life and death.

It all comes down to a paradox at the root of sport. In a May 1984 essay on competition in *Esquire*, George Leonard wrote: 'The worthy opponent is integral to the play, not an enemy but a co-conspiritor. The conspiracy is revealed in the word "compete" itself, which comes from two Latin roots, *com* and *petere*, "to seek together". In this light competition may be seen as a secret form of co-operation.' This thought is the basis of the words Australia's Team of the Century rugby league coach, Jack Gibson, often expressed when counselling a team against what he called 'cheap shots'. 'You wouldn't have a game unless you had an opposition', Jack drawled. Leonard noted a paradox at the root of competition: 'to elicit the most out of any game, one must play all out to win, yet at the same time not let an obsession with winning ruin one's pleasure in the game.' Cheating and cheap shots and lack of recognition for the opposition is an outgrowth of obsession with winning.

So back to the cricket. Ponting and his team inflamed their own nation because they did not acknowledge the losing team at the end of the gripping Sydney Test match. Most of the fury would have evaporated if a few of the Australians had wandered over and said to the Indians, 'Bad luck. You were stiffed. You should have got a draw out of that.' Ponting's second obligation, after celebrating with his team, should have been to extend some compassion to the Indians but, instead, he gesticulated defiantly to the commentary box where Channel Nine's Tony Greig had earlier suggested Ponting had left his declaration too late.

The Australian team's unbridled joy was understandable. Their mind-set had been locked into the inevitability of a draw—no other outcome seemed possible. A draw meant they would not have equalled the record for cricket's longest winning streak, sixteen successive Test match victories by an Australian team. But then came three sudden wickets by Michael Clarke—a part-time bowler. The outpouring of emotion was volcanic.

Still, their behaviour earlier in the match exposed a suspicion we have long felt about our national team: they are the quintessential bullies—they can give it but they can't take it. Their behaviour, both individually and collectively, deteriorates when their supremacy is challenged. Charges of hypocrisy were manifold, particularly on the last day of this Test. Wicketkeeper Adam Gilchrist, the saintly one who earned plaudits by walking in a semifinal against Sri Lanka in a World Cup match, calmly conspired to dismiss Indian middle-order batsman Rahul Dravid off the bowling of Symonds. Dravid was ruled to have deflected a ball, even though his bat was behind his pad. Surely none of the Australian team really thought Dravid was out? Gilchrist's predecessor, Ian Healy, explained the rationale to viewers from the commentary box. He said he had tended to appeal when he thought the batsman was out or when he thought the umpire might give him out.

Ponting, who had previously reached an agreement with the Indian captain to take the fielder's word on catches, justified his support for Michael Clarke's claim on a dubious low catch to dismiss the highly rated Sourav Ganguly by recalling a ball he volunteered had been grassed earlier in the Test. While Ponting would be expected to take the word of a team mate, it should also be pointed out that his earlier charity came when Australia's supremacy was not being challenged. Furthermore, Clarke's honesty surely must have been compromised by his earlier failure to walk when he edged a ball to first slip.

Most of the debate focused on Symonds, who snicked a ball and went on to score 162 not out. The following day's headline in *The Australian* captured the confused ethics: 'Hero Symonds: I was out on 30.' The Queenslander admitted he should have been out on the first day of the Test. 'I was very lucky. I was out when I was 30 and given not out,' he told a press conference. 'That's cricket, though. I could tell you about some bad decisions as well. That's the game. It's one of those things.' Former cricketers lampooned Symonds' honesty and even some of the media, who are forever railing about duplicity, dubbed his remarks ingenuous.

So what was Symonds expected to do? Lie? Okay, he undermined the credibilty of the umpire, Bucknor, who was of course later sacked—but not for incompetence according to the ICC; just in order to take some heat out of the explosive situation. The public didn't buy the ICC's line and perceived that the mighty rupee had purchased a sacrificial lamb. Nor did the public cop Symonds' claim that an Australian need not walk because the occasional poor decision is part of the game. For a start, it contradicted Ponting's argument that a fielder's word should be the final statement on a disputed catch. Surely, if a player is dishonest about nicking the ball, why should we imagine he is telling the truth about grassing it?

This episode neatly summarises the sport–business condundrum: either we play cricket for the sport, in which case we walk and don't need umpires, or we play for money, in which case we stay at the pitch and need umpires and all the technology available. And this exposes yet another inconsistency: is it fair on the umpires to give TV viewers and fans at the ground the benefit of instant accuracy through technology but deny such access to the decision makers? Yet when it was put to Channel Nine sports boss Steve Crawley that technology—such as 'snickometers', the 'hot spot' and 'Hawk Eye'—could be used to assist umpires, Crawley said he hated the idea of TV becoming the adjudicator of cricket matches and he questioned the accuracy of the new technology. Then why use these gimmicks if they give fans a false picture of the play? Ponting certainly agreed with Crawley, arguing that in the matter of low catches, neither technology nor the umpire's eye is superior to the word of the fieldsman. However, his agreement with the Indian captain to accept the fieldsman's word on catches collapsed because of the blatant hypocrisy in Sydney.

A new video review system was used two years later for the Australia–West Indies series. A batsman who believed he was incorrectly given out, or a fielding captain who believed a not-out decision was incorrect, could ask a video umpire for a review, with each team allowed two unsuccessful challenges per innings. However, at the end of the three Test series, won 2–0 by Australia, the umpire referral system had attracted controversy and confusion, with both captains agreeing it could be exploited by players. Two catches were claimed, only to be quickly overturned on review, but in the Perth test the third umpire ignored the evidence of the hot spot technology, which indicated a ball had not touched the bat, and backed the original decision of the field umpire to give the batsman out. The system also exposed cricket to the charge it is not a team game, particularly when desperate out-of-form batsmen use up the team's challenges to try and overturn decisions and improve their averages.

The SCG charge of racism against Harbhajan, laid by Ponting, also infuriated the Indian team. Symonds protested it was the second time the Sikh spinner had called him a monkey and that he had two months earlier complained about it after a one-day match in India. Judge Hansen certainly believed Symonds started the fight, referring in his judgement to an earlier agreement the two would not abuse each other on the field. 'This was initially breached by Mr Symonds' provocative abuse', Judge Hansen wrote.

The Indians displayed some duplicity of their own. They initially protested that the word monkey was a term of endearment on the subcontinent, as in 'you little monkey', but later claimed Harbhajan did not use the word. Furthermore, TV footage of the match in India clearly showed sections of the crowd taunting Symonds by scratching their armpits, simulating a monkey. The match referee believed the Australian's story and Harbhajan was initially suspended for three matches. But why would you believe anything the Australian team said they heard when they don't hear their own snicks and appealed when the opposing batsman was clearly not out? Furthermore, to the Indians it was a case of Australia benefitting from an anti-racism code when, in the eyes of many international players, the Aussies have been cricket's great racial abusers over the past 60 years. The Indians felt they were victims of a cultural lag.

Just as Australia wanted to beat England between the wars to show the mother country we could do more than produce wool and wheat, India craved recognition in the post-colonial era. But Harbhajan's ultimate escape also exposed one of the great truisms of sport: if there is a choice between the stuff-up theory and the conspiracy theory, go for the stuff up. The ICC, with weeks to prepare the documents for Harbhajan's appeal, did not provide the correct information about the Indian's involvement in previous breaches to Judge Hansen. The behind-closed-doors barrage of abuse by ICC CEO Malcolm Speed to his staff is unprintable. A female ICC lawyer had misread an email providing Harbhajan's past record. Fortunately, the media never became aware that she is a Hindu, saving the debacle from being blown at this time into a conspiracy theory. The email sent from London to her in Dubai could have been presented better, or she could have taken better care reading it, but she was mortified when she realised the implications of her stuff up. One of Harbhajan's past offences was committed under an old code of conduct and not included in the ICC database. A more serious recent offence was overlooked because more than one player was convicted and the entry on the database was made under another player's name. Judge Hansen later wrote in his judgement, 'Mr Singh can feel himself fortunate that he has reaped the benefit of these database and human errors'.

Judge Hansen also criticised the legalistic language of the player's code of conduct. Players seek resolution and crave certainty; weasel words are for lawyers. Eight months after Harbhajan escaped a meaningful sanction in the Adelaide Federal Court room, Symonds was being sent home from Darwin after failing to report to a team meeting because he was out fishing. Some media said the all-rounder's mind was elsewhere: he had not forgiven his own officials for convincing him and three of his team mates to downgrade the initial charge against Harbhajan to one of verbal abuse. Others said he felt abandoned by officials who were more interested in kowtowing to the rupee than protecting their own.

The truth is Symonds was troubled by an alcohol problem and preferred to fish than attend a meeting. He had 'moved on', to use the current vernacular, having arranged for the overland transport of his fishing boat from Brisbane to Darwin. Furthermore, he kowtowed to the rupee himself: he was the highest-paid player in the Indian Premier League. Player–official relations aside, evidence that the cricketers of both nations were still at war came with Gilchrist's autobiography, *True Colours*, released nine months later while Australia was playing India in India. Gilchrist, who had retired from international cricket, questioned the integrity of of India's most revered cricketer, Sachin Tendulkar.

The former Australian wicketkeeper suggested the Indian batsman changed his evidence at the Adelaide hearing to help Harbhajan escape the charge. Tendulkar was batting with Harbhajan when the Australians were convinced they heard the spinner call Symonds a monkey. Gilchrist described Tendulkar's evidence in his book as 'a joke', saying the batsman initially testified he had not heard what Harbhajan said but at the appeal claimed it was a Hindi word which could have sounded like monkey to Australians.

Yet Judge Hansen told the Melbourne sports law forum he found Tendulkar a very credible witness. 'In the Singh case, I was required, firstly, to determine whether the terms "monkey" or "big monkey" were used', Hansen said. 'By the time the matter reached me, it must be stressed that the evidence and the approach by those advising Singh was quite different than what occurred in front of the match referee. The additional evidence that was available to me and not the match referee included video footage from every camera on the ground with the commentary and sound, other than that from the stump microphone, removed. Although I question why this was not made available to the match referee, in this particular case it was of great significance. The match referee had found that Sachin Tendulkar was not in a position to hear what was said. In reality the video proved conclusively that he was standing next to Singh and was closer to him than anybody. At the appeal he proved an impressive witness.'

When Gilchrist's quotes sped around the cricket world, Harbhajan came to Tendulkar's defence. He said Indian players didn't share cricket's adulation of Gilchrist, saying, 'We don't respect him'. But nor is Harbhajan—who is nicknamed 'The Turbanator' and has a history of misbehaviour that is serially ignored by India's Board of Control—respected by the Aussies. Australia's opening batsman Matthew Hayden called him 'an obnoxious weed'. In his book Gilchrist said 'cultural differences' explained much of the problems between the teams, saying, 'In the Australian mentality, we play it hard and we then shake hands and leave it all on the field. Some of our opponents don't do it that way. Sachin Tendulkar, for instance, can be hard to find for a changing room handshake after we have beaten India. Harbhajan can also be hard to find.' Yet the one great disappointment to many Australians at that SCG Test was the disregard our team showed the Indians when they won the improbable match. In this case, post-match handshakes were hard to find.

Australia's cricketers had attended seminars in the lead-up to the Test series against India, listening to Cricket Australia telephonists recite the negative calls the organisation received after boorish displays in the field by the national team. Perhaps they listen but don't hear. On the first day of the third Test in Perth, ten days after the conflagration in Sydney, Ponting, interviewed on Channel Nine by former Australian captain Mark Taylor, expressed surprise that so much had been made of 'minor' incidents, conceding that in retrospect, 'We could have done some things differently'. Judge Hansen alluded to this in the paper to the sports conference, saying, 'Players and administrators also need to recognise that in the court of public opinion, if you are adept at dealing it out, you must be able to take it when there is a reaction to your own behaviour. I think it was probably this factor that resonated with much of the cricket world in the wake of the second Test in Sydney and which appeared to come as a shock to at least some of the Australian team.'

Ponting's critics predicted this was a Test from which the captain, who occupies a post considered by some the second highest in the land, would never recover. Afterwards, he reminded some observers of President George W. Bush's vacuous, inert response when the Commander-in-Chief had been told of the September 11 attacks during his visit to a Florida elementary school. Ponting looked bewildered, even guileless. In India, down one Test, Australia was in a commanding position in the fourth and final Test with a chance of squaring the series and retaining the Border-Gavaskar Trophy. But Ponting, after being warned that, if the overrate became too slow, he would be personally fined and banned for one Test, opted not to use his fast bowlers and the match ended in another defeat.

To add insult to ignominy, Harbhajan took the last wicket. Australia had surrendered its position at the top of the cricket world and suffered its most humiliating series loss in twenty years. Ponting stood accused of putting his own interests above victory, escaping a suspension to play mighty New Zealand in Brisbane.

Yet there was a rank odour of hypocrisy about the criticism. The same commentators who had accused him of leading a merciless bovver-boy team in Sydney were now saying he should have gone for the jugular in India. The self-appointed guardians of the game, who had castigated him for having a fine disregard for cricket's canons at the SCG, were now blaming him for obeying its laws in India. But Ponting had allowed himself to become distracted, not keeping check of the overrate, semi-asleep at the steering wheel.

Australia then lost the series against South Africa at home and surrendered the Ashes in England.

Furthermore, two years after the SCG test, Australian players showed how easily the goodwill they had gained could be lost when another home series ended with them being reminded of their obligation to uphold the spirit of cricket. Four members of the Australian team were fined for bad behaviour during the series win over the West Indies. All rounder Shane Watson attracted widespread criticism for his undignified wicket celebration when he bounded up and down in the personal space of Chris Gayle after taking the wicket of the West Indies captain for 21 in the Perth Test. Gayle merely stood and contemplated his fate only to look up and witness Watson's fenzied screaming in his face. Watson subsequently refused to explain his behaviour on Channel Nine—the rights holder, which effectively pays his salary. Nor did Ponting's promise to raise the matter at the team meeting 'when we go down to Melbourne' satisfy fans.

The West Indies players weren't blameless, indulging in numerous sledges on the field. But they were aggrieved by what they perceived to be disproportionate punishment by the ICC. West Indies team manager, Joel Garner, was seething when asked what he thought of the sanctions imposed on the Australian and West Indies players under the behavioural code. 'I go back to *Animal Farm* days, George Orwell,' Garner said. 'They say all animals are equal and later in the same book, they say some animals are more equal than others. Maybe that applies in some cases.'

Nor had cricket's international body demonstrated proper leadership two years earlier in the wake of Bollyline, certainly in terms of handling protests. When it is convenient for one of the world's wealthiest organisations to be thought of as running a sport and not a business, it can make a quick adjustment to the rising ball and behave like a stingy amateur sport. Hansen revealed, 'In July [six months after the Singh hearing], I was approached to see if I could conduct some training with the match referees who were having an annual meeting in London. I had been in the UK but by then had travelled to the US. I said I would make time available if they could arrange to cover my expenses. The response was there was no money for that.'

How much has the game really changed? Wasn't it Australian captain Bill Woodfull who, during the Bodyline tour, when English captain Douglas Jardine knocked on the dressing room door to demand an apology for being sworn at on the field, turned to his team and asked with a poker face, 'Which one of you bastards called this bastard a bastard?' Name-calling went on even earlier, when W.G. Grace, the legendary English captain, called the Australian team 'a damned lot of sneaks' in 1878. The doctor eventually apologised, telling Dave Gregory, Australia's first Test match captain, 'I wish to let bygones be bygones. I apologise again, and express my extreme regret to Conway, Boyle and yourself, and through you to the Australian cricketers, that in the excitement of the moment I should have made use of unparliamentary language.' W.G. was the only man in the history of Test cricket to regularly try to remain at the crease when clearly bowled, yet he managed an apology.

Still, of all the rules broken during that wrenching Test, only one was in writing: captains have an obligation to report to the umpire and their team management cases of racial abuse. All the other significant breaches—refusing to walk and claiming false catches—were unwritten.

During the ensuing controversy, the credo, 'it's just not cricket', received plenty of airing. It's a cliché unknown in any other sport, a phrase which has entered the language and gone beyond the boundary fence to describe an action considered reprehensible. It refers to a level of behaviour which, while not illegal, is simply 'not on'.

Yet there have been ample examples of unacceptable behaviour by Australians since the Bodyline tour when Australian batsmen risked decapitation from England's fast bowlers. The larrikin Australian teams captained by the Chappell brothers in the 1970s and early 1980s breached sporting norms, including intemperate outbursts by Dennis Lillee at the WACA—in 1979, during an Ashes Test, hurling an aluminium bat and, in 1981, kicking Pakistani provocateur Javed Miandad. Lillee and wicketkeeper Rod Marsh also placed a bet on the 500–1 English during the 1981 Headingly Test—and pocketed £7500 when the Poms eventually won. That year a third Chappell brother, Trevor, dispatched an underarm delivery to Kiwi tailender Brian McKechnie to prevent him hitting a six to win the match. Greg Chappell ordered the underarm delivery, enraging McKechnie, who threw his bat away in protest. New Zealand Prime Minister Robert 'Piggy' Muldoon reacted by describing it as 'the most disgusting incident in the history of cricket', adding, 'it was fitting that the Australians were dressed in yellow'.

Cricket's greatest figure, Sir Donald Bradman, remained at the crease after he was allegedly caught in the gully in the first Test against England in Brisbane in 1946. He had scratched out 28 in his return to the game and went on to make 187, infuriating English captain Wally Hammond. By not walking, Bradman rescued his comeback and booked his place as captain of the 1948 Invincibles.

'It's not cricket' invokes an earlier golden age of the game when players glorified in the amateur ideal—everyone walked, nobody made false appeals, there was no sledging, plenty of post-match handshakes and the spectators behaved admirably. The trouble is this golden age never existed. Furthermore, its 'noble' objective was to entrench the noble class. It promoted the 'Gentleman versus Players' games that endured until 1962. Professional players were required to walk out a different gate to the amateurs.

The stories of W.G. Grace cheating are manifold and most Australian players can recite the case of the young bowler who once clipped W.G.'s off bail, only to find Grace replacing the bail and saying, 'They've come to see me bat, lad, not you bowl.' Nor were players lilywhite amateurs. In 1884 in England, Australia fielded with only nine players because the other two believed the English opposition were being paid too much. In seeking to resolve the impasse, Australia's Billy Barnes broke his hand on a brick wall while trying to punch his captain, Percy McDonnell.

Nor were spectators well behaved. In 1882 in Sydney, an Australian cricket umpire ruled the local hero Billy Murdoch run out. Over 2000 spectators invaded the pitch and attacked the English players, while their captain, Lord Harris, was thrashed with a whip. And if Australians were offended by the term 'monkey' in January 2007, imagine how Indians felt about being called 'dirty blacks' by the MCC who barred them from selection, solely on racist grounds. In those days the Committee of the Test Ground were responsible for selecting the home team and in 1896 Ranjitsinhji, the brilliant Sussex batsman, was blocked by the MCC committee, led by Lord Hawke, from playing for England in the first Test at Lords. However, 'Ranji', when chosen for the second Test at Old Trafford by the Lancashire committee, scored 62 and 154 not out, the latter innings described by some as still one of the greatest of Test history. An MCC member, Lord Home Gordon, praised Ranji's innings, prompting another MCC member to turn on him, spluttering that he should be expelled from the club for having 'the disgusting degeneracy to praise a dirty black'.

So, if one can argue little has changed in cricket in nearly 150 years, how can we claim it is now too much of a business to be a sport? What has changed is the collapse of the old credo, 'What goes on on the field, stays on the field', or the broader 'What goes on on tour, stays on tour'.

Today's cricket, with its vast global audience, attracts at least 26 television cameras to every match, with their slow-motion scrutiny, microphones and reporters' pencils sharpened for the post-game press conferences. Blame professionalism and the global entertainment industry. If players want big money, they should realise most of it comes from TV rights. TV networks will use their 'stump cam' to pick up a foul-mouthed expletive or, at a football match, zoom their camera into a ruck to reveal a player biting an opponent—anything to generate increased ratings.

Increased audience numbers mean higher advertising rates and therefore more money for TV rights. Yet many of the officials of both the amateur disciplines and the professional codes are incapable of administering this challenging new world. Like a deer in the headlights, blinking and befuddled, they are caught at the crossroads of the new demands of business and the old responsibilities of sport.

TWO

HIGHER

Shortly after the 1994 Winter Olympics in Lillehammer, Norway, I travelled to Moscow to join an Australian delegation meeting with Russian Olympic officials. Following Sydney's award of the 2000 Summer Olympics, the Russian and Australian Olympic Committees had signed a joint agreement under which athletes of both nations would share training facilities, such as Canberra's Australian Institute of Sport. Our small delegation consisted of an AOC official, two heads of state sports institutes in Australia, myself (representing the Australian Sports Commission) and two scientists from the AIS who were on a bizarre mission to find out about some rare bird shit the Russians were using as a sports nutrient. We met with the Russians at their Olympic headquarters and a translator was present. Their leader was Anatoly Kolesov, a short, bald, muscular man who had won a gold medal in Greco-Roman wrestling at the 1964 Olympics. After an exchange of niceties, the questions began.

Drugs were foremost on my mind. My ASC position had placed me on a subcommittee to liaise with scientists at the recently established Australian Government Analytical Laboratory at Pymble, the nation's first sports drug-testing facility. These dedicated men had worked in an information vacuum, where the drug testers were desperately trying to catch up with the drug users. The AGAL biochemists were actually ingesting drugs and testing their own urine to measure dosage levels that would be detectable on a mass spectrometer. Rather than be worried about testicular shrinkage or future heart and liver disease, these committed men appeared to be more concerned about what they called 'false positives'—where a positive reading is in fact wrong, resulting in an athlete being punished because of inexact science.

'False negatives' were also a problem in this early era of vial and error. Don Catlin, the leading drugs expert at the time and head of an IOC-approved laboratory in California, said he saw fourteen false negatives for every provable positive at his lab. Scientists recognised it was almost impossible to catch a female drug taker—because testosterone does not occur as naturally in women as men, it takes only a miniscule amount of the artificial product to elevate performance levels quite magically.

The US 100-metre and 200-metre champion, Florence Griffith-Joyner, had won both titles at the Seoul Olympics in 1988 in times not expected to be reached until 2014. 'Flo-Jo', as she was called, died a few years after Seoul of uncertain medical causes. But the male 100-metre Olympic champion, Canada's Ben Johnson, had tested positive in Seoul to an anabolic steroid. Johnson had earlier won the world championship in Rome but his times in training in South Korea had been down. Perhaps he panicked and took one too many vials or tablets of Stanozolol, the anabolic steroid of choice at the time.

Even before reaching the finish line in Seoul, Johnson pointed to the sky and then stared across at the vanquished; his face was a mask of ferocity as he looked contemptuously at the US's Carl Lewis. He was so hot-eyed, he seemed wired. And on the big screen was an astonishing time: 9.79 seconds—faster than any other human had achieved and faster than anyone else would run for almost eleven years afterwards. Later, after he had been disqualified and his gold medal passed to Lewis, his coach, Charlie Francis, defended Johnson against accusations that the steroid gave him an unfair advantage. Francis said, 'It's only cheating if no-one else is doing it', a clear imputation that everyone in that 100-metre Olympic final was fuelled by drugs.

Australian pentathlete Alex Watson had also been sent home from Korea—for failing a caffeine test. The IOC had lowered the acceptable caffeine level from fourteen micrograms per millilitre in Los Angeles in 1984 to twelve in Seoul. The Australian team doctor at the time said it would have been impossible to drink enough coffee to produce all the caffeine Watson had in his system. The IOC subsequently dropped caffeine from its banned list in 2004, but at the time no-one could be sure how many beans you could have in every cup.

There had been whispered reports in Lillehammer of Russian long-distance skiers blood doping. So what was the truth of all this? When did drug taking begin in the Soviet bloc? Was it true that the muscled Renate Stecher, the East German athlete who had robbed our Raelene Boyle of gold medals in the 100 metres and 200 metres in Munich, was chemically enhanced? Was she the Typhoid Mary of steroids—the one responsible for its spread?

When I asked a question of Kolesov, a round mound of the seemingly profound, the collective intake of breath from the Australian delegation sounded like a swift wind blowing through a forest. My question was simply, 'When did the Soviet Union first use performance-enhancing drugs with athletes?'; but it clearly ambushed my fellow Aussies who seemingly sucked all the oxygen from the room and sat stunned, fearful they would be rushed off to some Siberian gulag. The question was slowly translated into Russian, eliciting mumblings from their delegates, which prompted my compatriates to nod sympathetically in Moscow's direction, as if to say, 'He's not really with us'.

The former wrestler answered in Russian, punching out his words forcefully, using *nyet* frequently, prompting even more angst from my colleagues. But when his answer was finally translated into English, my 'comrades' began breathing again. He welcomed the question, explaining that the Soviet's first knowledge of steroids came from information gathered on American gymnasiums, where puny desk-bound clerks who had enrolled at the local YMCA were suddenly looking like they had stepped out of a Mr Marvel comic. Russian spies told them American bodybuilders, powerlifters and the Mr Universes were heavily into drugs. He insisted he had seen literature from the early 1960s, written by American doctors, encouraging drug use. American athletes were going from being Ben Hogan to Hulk Hogan. It was inevitable, he said, the practice would flow to Olympic athletes.

Kolesov's view of history does not accord with the American understanding of the birth of steroids. An American, Dr John Ziegler, introduced steroids to US athletes: but he claimed to have done so after attending a world weightlifting championship in Vienna in 1956. Dr Ziegler says he was told that anabolic steroids were responsible for the impressive performances of Soviet athletes. He subsequently began work with a pharmaceutical company to develop a synthetic testosterone derivative with enhanced tissue-building properties known as Dianabol. No-one at the time realised an apt advertising slogan for the drug could have been, 'Die young, Die strong—Dianabol'.

The face of American sports—not to mention its bulging biceps, shrunken testicles and acne-riddled backs—was to change forever. Steroids became the Wheaties of the bodybuilders. While it led to grotesquely muscled men in Mr Universe competitions, to the freakish physiques of American football's he-lions and to baseball home-run records that should have an asterisk attached, it also spawned a cold war in track and field. At a time when the United States and Soviet bloc were engaged in a race to see who had the biggest nuclear arsenal, a similar strategy was put into place to armour-plate both countries' athletes. Not every father is proud of his progeny—shortly before Ziegler died in 1983, he said, 'I wish I had never heard the word steroid'.

While insisting the United States started the drugs race, Kolesov admitted drug use had become rampant amongst athletes in the United Soviet Socialist Republic in the late 1960s. He also conceded abuse of stimulants, particularly amongst cyclists, had been a major problem. Yet even in the 1980s Soviet athletes from various sports had popularised the use of catheters, through which clean urine could be injected into their bladders, from where it could be expelled for testing. This procedure clearly required the co-operation of doctors—the catheter had to be coated with antibiotics to reduce the high risk of infection and a local anaesthetic had to be used to cut the 100 per cent chance of pain!

Kolesov insisted drug use in Russia was on the decline at this time but he also mentioned he had been appointed chef de mission of Russia's team to the 1996 Atlanta Olympics. He was determined to beat the United States on the medal table. 'We can't compare with the Americans in living standards but we can in sport', he said. He argued the IOC Medical Commission had taken an unrealistic stance on drugs, banning too many.

'Some of these drugs assist athletes with their training loads but because they are banned, the athlete is forced to use weak medicines,' Kolesov said. 'The IOC must distinguish between drugs which cheat and those that help.' But if a drug assists the athlete in returning to training earlier, is it performance-enhancing?

Still, Kolesov's view was one with which Australian cricketer Shane Warne would have sympathised over a decade later. Warne was banned for a year by Cricket Australia for using a diuretic on the banned list of the World Anti-Doping Agency (WADA) which took over the IOC's duties in 1999. Diuretics are prohibited because they act as masking agents, disguising steroids; but Warne said he took the drug to lose weight. It was not as if he was seeking an advantage on the cricket field—he simply wanted to lose weight for reasons of vanity. He did lie about the number of tablets used—obtained from his mother—prompting the zealous boss of WADA, Dick Pound, to put the excuse in the same category as, 'I got it off the toilet seat.' The Warne saga, a tempest in a pee cup, went through days of hearings—an unfolding drama that would make any TV reality show producer weep with envy.

The truth is there is still mass confusion and double standards about drugs, even though athletes must abide by a code of strict liability—a caveat emptor ruling that basically says they are responsible for anything entering their mouth. Yet an IOC study of over-the-counter products showed that 45 out of 240 manufactured in the United States tested positive for banned ingredients that were not listed on their labels.

It's difficult, as most coaches know, to force athletes to read fine print, particularly scientific language. Furthermore, athletes, particularly footballers, can also be victims of a tug-of-war for power between trainers and doctors. The old trainer who has been at the club longer than the rubbing tables winks at the impressionable player and gives him a tablet that makes greyhound dogs go faster, while the club doctor hands out a printed sheet of 100 banned drugs . . . and the coach pretends not to know the difference. Coaches are capable of doing a very fine impersonation of the three monkeys when it comes to drugs.

There are no secrets in the dressing room; no-one spends a penny for someone else's thoughts. Insults are the lingua franca of the room. Nothing is sacred. There are constant quips and barbs about the sudden increased musculature of a rookie, or a veteran's quick recovery from injury, or—in the case of recreational drugs—nicknames for the spaced out. Coaches cannot possibly miss these references, yet often ignore them. Few pry in the manner of American football legend, Vince Lombardi, who once asked a player with blood-shot eyes, 'Have you been abusing yourself, Marvin?' Similarly, athletes have shown a remarkable capacity to feign innocence when it suits. Warne pleaded ignorance to the tablets he took; he claimed he was gazing out the window (or text messaging) during Cricket Australia's seminars on drugs, even though he recorded high marks in the quiz given after the lecture.

Food supplements and diuretics are not just used by elite athletes. They promise something for everyone: Michelangelo muscles, instant energy, washboard abs, overnight weight loss. They appeal to the short-attention-span and instant-gratification generation. A further lure of supplements and pills is they cross gender lines, tapping into everyone's insecurities about their bodies. For boys, it's the allure of adding muscle, particularly bulging biceps; for girls, manufacturers target aerobic improvement and weight loss. So, for young athletes—told to check every powder they take, while their peers are free to follow the dreams conjured up by the sports supplement manufacturers—it's all a bit confusing and unfair. One group's feats are athletic, while the other's achievements are synthetic; only the athlete knows how much time it takes in the weight room to get the same muscle mass.

And who is to say the bird shit the AIS scientists searched for in Moscow didn't come out of a packet? This magic elixir was called Mumio and was dropped by birds only at altitudes above 2000 metres. The AIS scientists had been told about Mumio by swim coach Gennadi Touretski, a Russian who had coached Olympic champion Alexander Popov and the winning Russian 4 x 100-metre relay team at Barcelona two years earlier but later shifted to the AIS. Touretski's first important swim coaching job was in Moscow. He was hired to develop the most-talented male swim sprinters born in the USSR in 1965—and he later told the AIS scientists that Mumio had been refined at a sports supplement laboratory in Moscow.

Maybe Gennadi had been in his cups at the time he confided the magic powers of Mumio. An alcoholic, he drank too much vodka on a flight to Hawaii prior to the 1996 Atlanta Olympics and was arrested by air marshalls. The very pious and (then) bitchy Australian Swimming Coaches and Teachers Association voted him off the team to Atlanta but, following secret representations from some senior male swimmers, AOC president John Coates overruled them. Then, in the lead-up to the Sydney Games, Gennadi was in trouble again when he was arrested for driving under the influence of alcohol after celebrating his Australian citizenship. Again, the coaches voted him off the team and, again, Coates, as team chef de mission, interceded on his behalf, famously saying, 'We didn't select him as a driver'.

*

Alcohol, over time, has certainly caused more damage to athletes and coaches than performance-enhancing drugs; but it is legal and, furthermore, generates massive sponsorships to sport. The AFL is sponsored by brewer Carlton, as is the Australian cricket team; the Queensland rugby league team enjoys one of sport's longest-serving relationships with rival XXXX and the Wallabies are supported by Bundaberg Rum. Critics quite correctly ask how the AFL and Cricket Australia can continue to take millions of dollars from the nation's biggest brewery, yet work themselves into a frothy frenzy over the addiction of Brownlow medallist Ben Cousins to cocaine—another 'recreational drug'—and Warne taking diet pills so he could look svelte while on a tour promoting the wine he sponsors!

Athletes have been searching for an edge since the ancient Olympics. The Greeks ingested herbs and hallucinogenic fungi, and Roman gladiators swallowed strychnine, mixing this potent stimulant, which heightens awareness, with wine. (Insofar as alcohol can also act as a somnambulant, the mix of wine and a stimulant would appear to be a combination that cancels itself out. It's a little like the joke about the drug that is half aphrodisiac and half tranquilliser, based on the theory that 'if you don't get a fuck, you don't give a fuck.')

Strychnine, without wine, was recommended for runners in short track events by Sam Mussabini, the coach of the British gold medallist Harold Abrahams, made famous in the movie, *Chariots of Fire*. Famous World War II American General George 'Blood and Guts' Patton admitted taking cocaine while competing for the US pentathlon team at the Stockholm Olympics. Tour de France rider Tom Simpson, who died while high on amphetamines in the 1967 race, once summed up this attitude toward pills: 'If it takes ten to kill you, I'll take nine.' In 1984, 198 world-class athletes were asked if they'd take a pill that would guarantee them a gold medal, even if they knew it would kill them in five years. Fifty-two per cent said yes.

But, in the early 1990s, the chemists were well ahead of the testers. Up to then, of those athletes caught, most had seriously overdosed or had engaged in bizarre methods to avoid detection. In 1978, Belgian cyclist Michel Pollentier strapped a bag of clean urine to his armpit and used the tube to drip the urine from under his shorts into the collection cup. Tour de France officials became suspicious during the collection of samples when Pollentier began pumping his elbow in and out, as if playing the bagpipes. American athletes in Seoul had been told they could avoid detection for steroids by smearing motor oil on their hands and then peeing on their greasy hands, allowing the urine to drip into the receptacle. Over the following years, athletes tried to mask illegal drugs by using vinegar, cleaning fluid and detergent. In 1994, British shot-putter Paul Edwards tested positive for drugs, including clenbuterol, a masking agent used to fatten cattle. When he was hospitalised for a stomach ailment, doctors discovered he had tried to flush his system by consuming water and liver salts.

In Atlanta, where Kolesov's Russians hoped to overtake the Americans, nobody anticipated the sudden success in the pool of Ireland's Michelle Smith, who won three gold medals. I was in the press conference when she was asked some leading questions, including the role of her Dutch fiancé, a track-and-field athlete banned from competition for testing positive to steroids, in her training. She was truculent, almost defiant, in her responses, and then-US president Bill Clinton reportedly told her not to worry about 'all that crap' from the press. But in August 1998, Smith was banned for four years for tampering with a urine sample required for a random drug test. She had been caught 'red-urined'. Her sample was spiked with what one tester termed 'a lethal concentration of alcohol', perhaps Irish whiskey.

The Chinese women swimmers, with their V-shaped backs, also raised eyebrows in Atlanta. Massive ingestion of diuretics had helped four of them pass performance-enhancing drugs through their systems quickly. But the diuretics showed up in tests at the world championships in Perth and the swimmers were suspended. Days earlier, another Chinese swimmer, Yuan Yuan, had been sniffed out by an airport dog named Dinky and found with thirteen vials of human growth hormone in her bag. (I once interviewed an attractive female Chinese weightlifter who won a gold medal at the world championships in Melbourne. I asked her the secret of her success. Through a translator, she replied 'dry roots and honey'—I suddenly had a sexy lead to the story!)

American footballers were possibly the first to use prosthetic penises to pass clean urine. When a Minnesota Vikings running back was discovered by airport security wearing one of these devices, it acquired a nickname, the 'Whizinator', and two Californian men who sold these fake penises were convicted of conspiracy. The lifelike penis emits clean, warm urine and comes with its own little heating unit and a supply of Yellow River urine packs. A website described the Whizinator as 'an easy-to-conceal, easy-to-use urinating device with a very realistic prosthetic penis'. It came in a variety of skin-tone colours to cater for the range of ethnic types. The device gave rise to what was called the 'Whizinator Rule' in the NFL—their pee collectors attended training camps and knocked on players' doors before dawn, demanding immediate samples.

The BALCO Affair in the United States changed the whole direction of drug detection—afterwards, the authorities basically were forced to admit they would have to rely on methods other than testing to catch athletes in future. The Bay Area Laboratory Co-operative (BALCO) in Burlingame, California, was revealed to have produced THG, a designer steroid. Marion Jones won five medals at the Sydney Olympics but everyone seemed in awe of the way she had navigated the minefield of sudden fame with arresting grace. Even when it was revealed during the Games that her husband, shot-putter C.J. Hunter, had tested positive four times, no-one wanted to believe graceful, gentle Marion was taking performance-enhancing substances. But a coach anonymously sent samples of the BALCO product to authorities and Marion and her new partner, 100-metre record-holder Tim Montgomery, were quickly implicated. Montgomery never tested positive but he was banned for two years, had his record erased, and went to prison for cheque fraud and heroin trafficking.

When BALCO founder, Victor Conte, revealed Marion's alleged drug calendar, with all its coded notations, on network TV, some writers were reminded of *The Great Gatsby*, in which young Jay scheduled times for wall scaling, the study of electricity and the 'practice of elocution'. These pursuits, as far as Jay Gatsby was concerned, were the human development hormones of the day. But for today's highly competitive young men and women, vaingloriously chasing gold medals that can buy a dream home—the American hero in other words—the rules of play will always be open to adjustment.

Marion vigorously defended herself, despite Conte being her

official 'nutritionist' at the Sydney Games; she burned more calories trying to remain a US athlete than actually being one. She even changed coaches, bizarrely choosing Charlie Francis, the man who had tutored Ben Johnson! Her lawyers even boasted she passed a lie detector test, in which she was asked if she had ever taken performance-enhancing drugs. Wags joked the results of the polygraph did not count because they were wind assisted.

I found myself thinking about Marion when I climbed Mount Kilimanjaro with a group of friends in 2008. When you climb through the night, it helps to concentrate your mind if you pose yourself a puzzle. Kilimanjaro is nearly 6000 metres high and altitude sickness is a concern. But it's only two-thirds the height of Everest, the limit man can climb without the assistance of oxygen in cylinders. Was this ordained by God? Did he thrust that white fang up into the sky, making it the highest point on earth, beyond which no human can climb without the help of science? I found myself comparing Marion with Sir Edmund Hillary, the first man to climb Everest.

Hillary reached the summit with the use of oxygen despite being technically able to avoid it. Thousands have since followed, assisted by ever-improving equipment—lightweight, layered clothing; improved crampons; stronger, lighter ropes and a better understanding of altitude sickness. The tents in Hillary's day were made of canvas and oxygen was carried in cylinders that weighed twenty kilograms. Nowadays, with Everest base camp in risk of becoming a garbage dump with a steady file of moutaineers climbing to the top aided by high-tech gear, I concluded there was a sad irony in all this. The new wonders our scientists are creating in laboratories for our athletes and mountaineers merely serve to reduce the majesty of the natural world. In other words, the past's adventurers, such as Hillary, had become the present day's tourists; yesterday's milestones chronicled on *MovieTone News* are today's passing highlights on the internet.

I later learned no serious climber will now attempt Everest with the aid of portable oxygen. Two Europeans, Reinhold Messner and Peter Habeler, reached Everest's summit together in the 1980s without the use of oxygen. So, unless the serious mountaineer is attempting a difficult route, no self-respecting climber will carry it—otherwise, he would consider himself a tourist.

I remember attending a press conference in England when the Welsh rugby league player, Jonathan Davies, announced he was returning to rugby union. It was around the time rugby union had officially become professional. Davies was asked whether the fact rugby union players were now paid would halt the defections to rugby league. He said it would not because the best players would always want to test themselves in the tougher arena of league. It was not an answer that would please rugby purists, given their belief that theirs is the more mentally challenging code. But Davies was putting himself in the same category as Messner–Habeler: elite sportsmen will always seek challenges.

When Hillary climbed Everest, four minutes also appeared as the barrier to the mile. The time had withstood decades of human yearning and exertion. It was a figure that seemed so perfect—four laps, four quarter miles, four point 00 minutes. It seemed as if God had established it at the halfway mark of the twentieth century as man's limit—a gentle reminder of the natural order of things against the backdrop of the devastation of two world wars. It's an arrogant thought, given that the mile was only relevant to the world of imperial measurements. The 1500 metres was the distance of Europe. (When Ireland's Ron Delany won the 1500-metre gold medal at the 1956 Melbourne Olympics there was joy throughout the Emerald Isle, as comedian Brian Doyle remembers: 'Everyone is happy when Irish guys are miling.')

This was a time when the title 'world's fastest human' (the Olympic 100-metre winner) ran second fiddle to the mile and the 1500-metre champions. The four-minute mark—there was actually a thrill in the words 'four-minute mile'. It was the Holy Grail of athletics, similar to the sound barrier, something to be broken, possibly at great physical peril. The mark fell within a short time of Hillary conquering Everest and Australia's John Landy broke it again six weeks later. It was that pale-skinned explorer of human exertion, Dr Roger Bannister, who did it first on the drizzly afternoon of 6 May 1952 at the Iffley Road Track in Oxford, England. It became the day the clock was beaten, yet Bannister later reminded us, 'I have always said man will run the mile in 3.30, given the human body constituted as it is, with perfect training and perfect facilities'. He was passing on the torch to others, as Hillary did to Messner–Habeler.

Consider Bob Beamon's long jump at the 1968 Olympics. It was, in all respects, a jump weirdly perfect. He planted his foot precisely at the end of the board and came off it like a huge loose-limbed frog, his legs spread-eagled and his arms dangling. He had the maximum allowable two-metres-per-second assisting wind and gained optimum elevation by flying through the reduced density of the air of the high-altitude Mexico City. Even the physiologists who observed him exhausted afterwards were convinced he had somehow summoned the superhuman strength that ordinarily only comes to people in disasters. I was in Japan in 1991 at the world championships when Beamon's mark was bettered by fellow American, Mike Powell. There was something strange about the weather in Tokyo—a major typhoon loomed off the coast. On another evening three men broke the world record in the epic 100-metre sprint final and six ran under ten seconds with an allowable tailwind. Similarly, when Bannister broke the four-minute-mile record, the skies cleared five minutes before the race. Isn't there mystery enough in these record-breaking achievements, even in supernatural weather, without the intrusion of drugs?

Eventually, Marion Jones was jailed and authorities used her case to lobby for a lowering of the burden of proof for athletes suspected of steroid use. It sought to relax the criterion from 'beyond reasonable doubt' to 'comfortable satisfaction'. It all ended up sounding like a meal, which was what the US Olympic Committee made of it. US track-and-field athletes had been protected for years by the numerous appeals and the secretive nature of the arbitration process that followed positive tests. It was a system rooted in confidentiality and due process; a protocol long on fairness but sometimes short on commonsense. If the response from the authorities over the BALCO revelations sounded almost hyperactive, it was because the Americans were trying to undo decades of ill will, including whispers that some test tubes of the sainted Carl Lewis had gone missing at the 1984 Los Angeles Olympics.

The snickers of recognition—once reserved for supersized Eastern European women in the 1980s and for African men and Chinese women who shattered distance running records in the 1990s—have now been transformed into whispers of accusations against all. When Jamaica's Usain Bolt broke the men's world 100-metre and 200-metre records at the Beijing Olympics in 2008, we could not totally give of ourselves and surrender to the joy of the moment for fear we would be disappointed a few days later with the announcement of a positive test. Our response to records now is far more tempered. Cynicism is a painful substitue for awe. Only when Bolt bettered both times at the World Championships in Berlin a year later did some of us start to believe his times were the result of a longer stride and an unusually quick start for an athlete so tall.

American baseball was also caught up in the BALCO enquiry when two of its biggest stars, Barry Bonds and Jason Giambi, became the twin lightning rods in the storm of drug allegations battering America's most popular sport. Both men admitted using 'the cream', a testosterone-based balm rubbed into the skin, and 'the clear' (THG), a liquid steroid taken in drops under the tongue. The scandal reinforced a wide perception that baseball was powerless to prevent the use of performance-enhancing substances and reluctant to address the issue.

The sport's leaders were exposed as duplicitous, uncooperative and basically clueless. In one year (2003), 70 major baseball players failed anonymous tests for steroids when they knew they were to be tested. How many players had used steroids over the previous fifteen years when no tests were in place, and no repercussions involved? The American public certainly let the sport know what it thought: when Bonds was presented with an award at the 2004 World Series as baseball's best hitter, he was booed. He had eclipsed the home-run record of Babe Ruth, a pudgy hitter who lived on a diet of beer, hot dogs and staying out late with women. Many called for Bonds' records to have an asterisk attached.

If any event demonstrated the lengths to which athletes will go to win, it was the Sydney Paralympics, held shortly after the abled-bodied Games. Wheelchair track athletes sat on tacks and ball bearings, stuck themselves with pins, tied piano wire around their scrotums, or clamped off their catheters until their bladders were almost at bursting point. Because these athletes are paralysed, they suffered no pain but their sympathetic nervous systems went into overdrive, pushing up their blood pressures, activating their fight-or-flight adrenaline responses and improving their performances by as much as fifteen per cent. Wags joked that this was how the TV character 'Ironside' caught all the criminals! Or wondered who needed blood doping when they could have nut roping?

Ten weightlifters from nine countries tested positive for performance-enhancing drugs. But the real shock came a month after the Games when a Spanish magazine reported that fifteen members of Spain's paralympic team weren't *discapacitados* (disabled). The magazine author should know, he was one of the fifteen! He played in Spain's intellectually disabled basketball team, which romped away with the gold medal. That team contained ten players who were not intellectually disabled, including a lawyer, an engineer, some students and, of course, the journalist. The Paralympics require a player to have an IQ of 70 or less to be eligible for intellectually disabled competition, but the journalist said he was never tested.

The drug of choice for young athletes determined to build up body mass in order to perform better on the field, or to train harder, is human growth hormone. This substance is only detectable by a blood test within four hours of use. An athlete who injects himself at midnight and then retires to bed is unlikely to be woken by sample collectors at 2 am. In any case, most sports allow only urine tests, not blood sampling. Human growth hormone, available in most anti-ageing clinics, is also within the budget range of semi-professional athletes—a month's course selling for $600.

EPO (erythropoietin) has been the wonder drug for endurance athletes since the early 1990s. Urine tests reveal evidence of its use dating back only three days, meaning an athlete could use it four days before testing and be officially clean. For years, cycling's Tour de France has been less a movable feast than a movable pharmacy. Cycling authorities gave tacit acceptance to EPO's use by setting a level similar to octane content in petrol. Cyclists were permitted to use 'standard' fuel, but if they moved into the high-octane 'super' stuff, as some Tour de France leaders did after a day of poor times, they were caught. Athletes have also found another use for Viagra, which facilitates blood flow. They mix it in a cocktail with caffeine pills and pseudoephedrine to boost performance.

An investigation in Spain led to seven cyclists being suspended from the Tour de France (which could be named the 'Tour de Syringe') at a time when the new generation EPO was being used. Spanish police received a tip-off that a doctor was prescribing a drug called CERA to athletes and placed him under surveillance, including the use of wire taps. After gaining enough evidence for an anticipated prosecution, police entered the premises and confiscated patient records and seized labelled blood samples from a fridge.

The use of human growth hormone—described by Australia's then sports drugs boss, Richard Ings as 'an insidious form of doping, undetectable and dirt cheap'—has led to a diversion of resources to investigation, as opposed to testing. Half the budget of the Australian Sports Anti-Doping Authority is spent on detection. The Federal Government granted ASADA powers to obtain information via data sharing with federal and state police forces, customs, the Therapeutic Goods Administration and state medical boards. WADA lists eight violations, with only three dealing with positive tests. Tampering with drug protocols, trafficking, administration of a prohibited substance, even being caught with drugs in the athlete's possession are deemed to be an offence. WADA grants itself a catch-all violation—'failure to comply'—which bestows wide powers on all agencies. WADA has also reached an agreement with Interpol to share information. It ultimately hopes to introduce a biological passport that will monitor an athlete's biological parameters over years and so detect abnormal variations which could derive from doping. ASADA has taken a similar course and stores urine samples in a giant vessel, called 'the tank', for re-examination in years to come when science may have found a test for an undetected drug. The IOC will continue to test Beijing Olympic samples for another eight years.

Had this 'stale bottle of piss' been in operation in the 1970s, 'our Raelene' may have had a couple of golds. ASADA's comprehensive powers also include the ability to cross-check credit card details and emails that come under its notice. 'We have IT code crackers', Ings once told me, claiming his organisation would become the equivalent of business's anti-competition watchdog, a further reference to the link between big-time sport and business. 'We will do what it takes', Ings said. 'We want to be the ACCC of sport. Just as ACCC protects the honest businessman, we seek to guarantee the honest sportsperson has a drug-free level playing field. Our mission is to put ourselves out of business. We'll know we've been successful when we are no longer necessary.'

How do domestic sporting bodies, international federations, or agencies know when they have been successful? Do twenty positives a year in a sport with one thousand athletes mean it has a problem? Does one positive test mean you are winning because you have caught only one? Or does it mean you are losing because you haven't caught a hundred? The main problematic zones with drugs are top-grade players taking so-called social drugs and fringe players using performance-enhancing substances, plus players taking drugs in order to come back from injury quicker. Having a successful anti-doping code usually depends on how many tests are administered and whether they are for performance-enhancing drugs, or social drugs, or both. Many people don't know the difference, including former Prime Minister John Howard who was questioned in a door-stop interview at the height of the AFL's 'social drug' crisis. Howard, like many, was confused whether certain drugs were banned under the WADA code or the sport's voluntary code.

For years the AFL boasted it didn't have a drug problem, compared to the NRL. Historically, however, the AFL commissioned ASADA to conduct only half as many tests for performance-enhancing drugs. Furthermore, rugby league players were tested out of competition, whereas the AFL swabbed only on match days. This meant an NRL player could be tested for cocaine at a mid-week training session, while an AFL player would only be swabbed immediately following a game. Not surprisingly, rugby league recorded three positives to illicit sustances over the decade during which these 'party' drugs became widespread, while the AFL had none. But then along came the West Coast Eagles' Brownlow medallist Ben Cousins—arrested in Perth, he was escorted unsteadily to a police car, during which his bare torso revealed a Ned Kelly 'Such Is Life' tattoo.

The AFL was forced to admit it had a problem. Despite being a self-confessed addict, Cousins had never recorded a positive. For years his behaviour in Perth had been bizarre and his wind-up whooping celebrations on the dais after his team won the AFL premiership suggested he was on something higher than the joy of winning. He was as overt about drug use as American baseballer Tim Raines in the 1980s, who slid head first into a base so as not to disturb the vial of cocaine in his back pocket. Even when Cousins was exposed, the AFL persisted in boasting it was the only sporting organisation in Australia to test for social drugs on non-match days. Yet NRL club Broncos permit themselves to test their players unannounced at any time of the day or night, across the entire week, or 24/7 in the shorthand language of today. The Broncos conducted 280 tests in the year Cousins was not caught, more than half the 500 tests the AFL administered on its list of 640 players.

Most players who use the popular social drugs—cocaine, ecstasy and ice—take them in the post-match period when they are celebrating or needing a lift after a defeat. These drugs are cheaper than alcohol—an 'ekky' costs $20—and a player can socialise all night, accompanied by only a bottle of water. (Some nightclubs once refused to sell water—not because they were being responsible but to extract some alcohol money from the player's pocket.) Furthermore, drugs don't stack on the kilograms as alcohol does, and most clubs insist players weigh in at least once a week. Nor does the player wake up with a hangover. But, most importantly, players know these drugs leave the system within 24 hours, meaning they are unlikely to be caught if their next test is a week away, the day of their next match.

When Wendell Sailor, then playing rugby union for New South Wales, tested positive to cocaine following a match-day swab, he was shocked—particularly because he was partying with another high-profile footballer who wasn't caught. Cocaine enhances performance but 'Dell' insisted he did not take it for this purpose. And he was telling the truth. He had become an habitual user and the cocaine, taken five days earlier, was still in his system. So Dell received a two-year ban for taking a performance-enhancing substance, although the penalty would have been lower if rugby union had had a recreational drugs policy in place, similar to the AFL and NRL.

Like Cousins, rugby league's most prominent drug user, Team of the Century halfback Andrew Johns, never tested positive. He admitted to 'running the gauntlet'—gambling the drug testers would not arrive at an early-morning training session following the previous night's game. But Johns' heavy drug use came during a time the NRL had delegated out-of-competition testing of social drugs to the clubs. The new WADA code, introduced to provide uniformity across countries and sport, did not require sporting organisations to run out-of-competition testing for social drugs. So the NRL, which was the first code in Australia to integrate a performance-enhancing drug policy with an illicit substances code—on one occasion testing every player in a 24-hour blitz—devolved the responsibility for social drugs to its clubs. Guess what? Johns' Newcastle club was one of only two which didn't test. When you've got the best player in the world on your books, why deprive yourself of his services via a lengthy ban? Furthermore, the Knights have always struggled financially and testing is expensive. You get the impression that if Joey had tested positive to marijuana, the Knights would have listed him on the injury report as 'doubtful man!' An entrenched club culture is hard to change. Despite the Knights embracing testing in the post-'Joey' years, their officials were shattered when two of their top players were charged by police late 2009/early 2010 for trafficking drugs.

WADA demonstrates a degree of hypocrisy by not enforcing out-of-competition testing for social drugs. There are three issues used to justify sports conducting drug tests: cheating, danger to health and the role-model argument. By not insisting sports conduct out-of-competition testing for illicit social drugs, WADA is effectively abrogating responsibility for athletes' health and sport's role in setting an example to impressionable youth.

Some of the most professional sports in the world occasionally show a reluctance to punish sportspeople testing positive to what they euphemistically call 'recreational' drugs. A French tennis player successfully convinced authorities his positive test came from one kiss with a cocaine-using female. Maybe WADA doesn't wish to burden cash-strapped sports with additional costs but when the NRL finally decided to introduce a uniform system of testing across all clubs, this coincided with an announcement by ASADA that it would increase the charge of a full screen test by 45 per cent. So, at $950 a sample, the NRL was forced to admit it may have to halve the number of mandated tests.

The dangers to health from drugs have never been announced as prominently as the warnings you see on cigarette packets. The early advertisements for mail-order muscles in magazines showed pumped-up bodybuilders—illusory images of masculinity and virility from which hanged, metaphorically and ironically, their steroid shrunken testicles. My wife, Elaine Canty, a former ABC broadcaster and lawyer, was the first to document in the Australian media the harmful effects of steroids. She interviewed a female shot-putter who spoke in a deep voice and referred to hair on her bum and a clitoris shaped like a small penis. Yet the major sports failed to seize upon these admissions to alert athletes to the list of complications after using steroids and what fool's gold they are.

The most serious adverse side-effect is liver dysfunction leading to liver cancer. For males, there's also a reduction in the size of testes, diminution in sperm quality and the loss of sex drive. For women, there's the appearance of facial hair, deepening of the voice and enlargement of the clitoris. The East German drug regime involved up to 10,000 athletes, including a number of women who later gave birth to children who were blind or had club feet. When observers noted that members of the 1976 East German women's swim team to the Montreal Olympics had particularly deep voices, their coach unashamedly replied, 'We have come here to swim, not sing'.

This attitude is typical of those who would abandon all drug testing. The arguments traditionally used to allow a free-for-all are: there is no scientific proof drugs enhance performance; athletes have a right to take their own risks; the drug police will never catch all the users, so give up. Another argument sometimes advanced is that because our genes decide our body chemistry we should be free to modify that chemistry in order to exploit our full genetic potential. Yet the fact remains, it is unacceptable in medical ethics to risk the serious side effects of drugs unless treating a serious disease. This ethic should outlaw doping, whether it enhances performance or not.

Hypocrisy over drug testing is not the exclusive domain of clubs, sports, international federations and agencies. When the AFL in late 2008 gave Cousins permission to play—after a twelve-month ban for 'bringing the code into disrepute'—the announcement led most Melbourne radio bulletins for days, relegating the global financial crisis to second-tier news. Three clubs expressed interest in Cousins but two withdrew because of pressure from sponsors. Richmond was left as the single suitor and a digitally created photo of Cousins wearing a Tigers' jumper made the lead page of both Melbourne daily newspapers. It was not as if their front-of-the-jumper sponsor, electronics chain Dick Smith, needed additional name recognition in the marketplace, but there was a report that a wealthy restaurateur, who had previously played for Richmond, would become a subsidiary sponsor if Cousins was signed. So while sponsors at other clubs were afraid of the damage Cousins would do to them in the marketplace, Richmond profited from the increased recognition value of their sponsorships and the 4000 additional club members who subsequently signed up. Super Rugby club Western Force also expressed interest in Cousins. But the Perth-based club had lost its main sponsor Firepower—a company that conned people into believing it had produced a pill which, when mixed with water, became petrol. Perhaps they hoped the 'pill popping' Cousins would deliver another backer.

Cousins was in a position to profit from the drama. A documentary has been made about his volatile career—a TV package with the potential to ignite an eager bidding war amongst broadcasters in the AFL-obsessed southern states. AFL executive commissioner Andrew Demetriou once told a colleague that his aim was to supply the media with one major story a day. Cousins made his job easier and the AFL strung out the midfielder's return to football, making pronouncements ahead of the national draft and then the pre-season draft, before the Tigers acquired him.

The saga did not end with TV footage showing excited young Richmond fans greeting him at Melbourne airport, ahead of his first training session, in a black-and-gold jumper. The same day, a court heard he had been associating with a gangster charged with ordering the execution of a drug trafficker. The AFL imposed strict conditions on Cousins—he was required to submit to three urine tests a week and provide four hair samples a year. His immediate reaction was to shave down and have a full body wax, meaning those hair follicles were going to be hard to find! It also produced the headline in *The Age* newspaper: 'Cousins on notice over hair length.' Thirty years ago, the same headline in Sydney would have referred to long-haired Eastern Suburbs rugby league players being barred from entering their Bondi Junction Leagues Club.

Cousins' 'control order conditons' were probably less onerous than those imposed on convicted terrorist David Hicks, yet the AFL action exposed the hypocrisy of their three-strikes policy. AFL players are effectively given two free get-out-of-jail cards before they are banned but Cousins had never tested positive. The AFL admitted at this time that several unnamed players were currently on two strikes, yet were being allowed to play, with possibly two contributing to Hawthorn's win in the 2008 grand final. In other words, they were on two strikes more than Cousins who was banned from playing that year. Yet the AFL refused to concede their drug policy was flawed, or admit there was confusion whether they were motivated by care for Cousins' welfare, or concerned he would relapse if allowed back on the field. 'World-class medical advice' is the reason cited by the AFL to justify the three-strikes policy, arguing that rehabilitation is more important than punishment. Addicts recover best when they receive anonymity, according to the AFL.

But name and shame is a powerful deterrant, as USA Track & Field, the governing body for athletics in America, eventually discovered. Being named as a drug user in the media is the modern equivalent of doing time in the stocks in the town square—being mocked and pelted with rotten tomatoes. Marion Jones' fall from grace was a salutary lesson. In any case, when the AFL finally do announce the name of a drug user—after his third strike—it would suggest rehabilitation has failed and he is presumably at his most fragile point, psychologically. Furthermore, the AFL policy of keeping the name of a player testing positive a secret from everyone at his club, except the medical officer, has been criticised by club doctors who say it would assist a player's rehabilitation if non-medical officials, such as coaches, were also informed. Nor does the AFL allow clubs to engage in supplementary testing. West Coast Eagles coach John Worsfold claimed club tests might have provided more intelligence on what was an almost epidemic-sized problem in Perth. Keeping a lid on the number of positives is an effective way of denying you have a problem.

Compounding all the confusion, duplicity and double standards over sportspeople and drugs is our hypocrisy over punishments meted out to our own athletes, as opposed to overseas competitors. When swimmer Sam Riley tested positive, her fiercely patriotic Brisbane supporters all agreed she had taken a headache tablet given to her by her coach, extracted from the bottom of his training bag for such an early-morning emergency. How dare anyone put the cupid-faced Sam in the same class as those Chinese swimmers with acne-scarred skin! Similarily, would the media have given a sympathetic run to Schapelle Corby, jailed in Bali for bringing marijuana into the country, if she were less attractive?

We celebrate international musicians who have written top-of-the-chart songs under the influence of chemicals, yet savage East German athletes of the same era. We wink at the Beatles 'Lucy in the Sky with Diamonds', knowing it refers to LSD, while excusing the 'fab four' for drug use. The English poet Samuel Taylor Coleridge wrote the first verse of *Kubla Khan* while in an opium trance, yet, when woken by his landlady, he could not replicate its magic in the second verse. Politicians and moral crusaders do not mention poets and artists when they use the role-model argument to support drug bans. Perhaps acid-induced, performance-enhanced rock musicians with their overdose deaths, bizarre lifestyles and their high salaries are someone else's role model!

I lived opposite the artist Brett Whiteley for a time, a couple of years after I finished coaching St George. When people discussed his most expensive works at the pub, they would giggle about his heroin use and how it contributed to his greatest works. Yet the same people were appalled when a random drugs test at South Sydney rugby league club resulted in positive tests for marijuana. There appears to be an inconsistency between the public's relaxed approach to an artist taking performance-enhancing substances and the public's expectation that footballers should be punished for taking a substance that diminishes performance. Surely the argument that footballers are more effective role models than artists shouldn't make any difference.

It's hard to escape the notion that the authorities—other than officials such as the consistently hard-lined but pragmatic Coates (his relaxed attitude to alcohol notwithstanding)—have failed athletes. They have obfuscated over drugs for a long time, doing their best impression of ostriches. Players' union bosses have been willing accomplices, declaring they really are concerned about the health of their players, not the health of players' pay packets, despite blocking steroid testing or opposing a three-strikes policy. You get the impression that if players start dying, their response will be to do a deal with a florist shop.

Should we really be surprised if the world's most celebrated gold-medal-winning athlete is revealed as taking performance-enhancing drugs? Our society is driven by the principle of self-improvement. Look at the bestseller lists—they are all about a better diet, a more efficient budget, a cleaner house, improved grooming, a more tranquil frame of mind, even a more obedient pet. Our TV shows rely heavily on the makeover fantasy—the sudden renovation of a house, a garden, a restaurant. There's nothing that can't be enhanced (whether it is breasts, vocabulary, hearing or erectile function) or stapled (stomachs) or tucked (wrinkles) or lasered (eyes). So why should we be shocked when our finest athletes—with their truly outsized ambitions and vanity—seek chemical opportunity?

Okay, unlike Jay Gatsby's wall scaling and elocution, it's illegal and unfair, and this new pharmaceutical frontier ahead of us could be deadly. But what if a day dawns when performance additives are as safe as Nature's Way vitamins, and athletes seduce themselves into believing they are no more unfair than access to better coaching, training facilities and superior competition? Medical practitioners will counter this by pointing to side effects—some potentially unknown—and, in any case, there's still the cheating angle. Furthermore, do we want spectators to attend athletic festivals where the only real competition is between the chemists? Do we want a world where only the rich nations win because the poor can't afford the laboratories or the importation of the subtances that make them go faster, or leap higher, or lift heavier weights? The same argument—addressed later in this book—applies to the use of high-tech swimsuits, carbon-fibre bicycles and sophisticated yachts. Surely, it's more than a coincidence poor African countries do badly in swimming, cycling and yachting at Olympic Games.

None of the philosophical arguments against the use of drugs cut much slack with the competitors. The one educational campaign about drug use most neglected is the one that might well be the most effective: sending athletes the message of the danger to health. Officials can test athletes until their cup runneth over but they will find deaf ears with the role-model argument. Character, self-respect and decency in sport will always be discarded in favour of the pursuit of perfection. It's hard to feel guilty winning the Tour de France when you're pursued by similarly chemically enhanced contenders.

Coaches can make a difference. Athletes have great trust in their mentors. A coach who warns of the harmful effects of steroids and stimulants is sending a message he cares for the athlete and not his own win–loss record. But he's wasting his time if he philosophises about cheating, illegalities and the role-model argument.

THREE 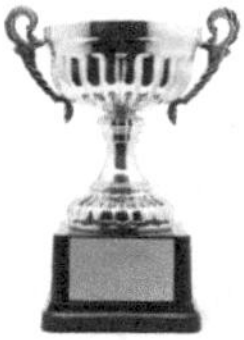 RICHER

When Sydney radio stations reported in July 2008 that Canterbury Bankstown player Sonny Bill Williams had secretly walked out on his team mates to catch a plane to Paris to play rugby union for a French club, the NRL's most intransigent, insular club finally realised Fortress Belmore was no more. The Bulldogs had contempuously defied accusations of salary cap abuse and sexual assault, deluding themselves into believing that what didn't kill them made them stronger. But the flight of their best player to another code catapulted them into the world outside the southwestern suburbs of Sydney. They finished the season as wooden-spooners, a rare position for a club that had been one of rugby league's top performers over the previous 40 years. Even their coach, Steve Folkes, was forced to bow to globalisation by securing a job with the West Indies cricket team as their strength-and-conditioning coach.

A few months earlier in England, I witnessed another confrontation over globalisation, the buzzword that describes the ever-expanding exchange of goods and services across national borders. I was with NRL premiers, the Storm, on a visit to the north of England to play a World Club Challenge match against Super League premiers, Leeds Rhinos. We bussed up to Liverpool to watch a soccer game against Middlesborough at Anfield and, after the match, the son of Tom Hicks, the Texan co-owner of the local team, was showered with beer and spat at in the Anfield pub where the Liverpool club had been originally founded.

Hicks Senior also owned baseball's Texas Rangers and American ice hockey's Dallas Stars. His partner, fellow American George Gillett Jnr, owned the Montreal Canadiens ice hockey team and also had interests in NASCAR racing. Hicks' father had fallen out with Gillett, who was under financial pressure, and at this time Dubai International Capital, the investment arm of the Dubai Government, was reported to be interested in owning the Merseyside club. Tom Hicks Jnr, besuited and surrounded by minders, had provocatively stepped out of a silver 4WD and into The Sandon pub on Anfield Road; entering the less noisy middle bar, he ordered a pint of lager for himself and soft drinks for his security team. But when his suit and his likeness to his father gave him away, he began fielding questions about his father's plans to sell the club to an Arab group. Gradually the approaches became more indignant and the crowd started to sing anti-American protest songs. As insults flew, Hicks found himself drenched by a pint.

There's nothing novel about owners falling out over debts involving football clubs. The friendship between businessman Peter Holmes à Court and actor Russell Crowe, co-owners of the NRL's Rabbitohs, cooled when the spendthrift Peter asked the tight-fisted Russell to tip in a few million to cover the club's debts. Developer Max Delmege and health industry businessman Scott Penn, co-owners of the NRL's Sea Eagles, fell out over their plans to buy the Manly Leagues Club.

Nor is there anything unusual about foreign ownership of English soccer clubs, or indeed those proprietors also having interests in franchises of other sports. Increasingly, the twenty English premier league clubs are falling into the hands of Americans, Russians, Arabs, even Icelanders. Young Hicks was a victim of the passion, sometimes self-recrimination, fans feel when their club slips from local control.

In the same way that Liverpool fans had long resented the loss of their entire club to foreigners, Bulldogs' fans in Sydney felt impotent to stop the departure of their best player to a French billionaire who made his fortune publishing comic books. On the other hand, the International Rugby Board (rugby union) wasn't about to take action to support the Bulldogs over the Sonny Bill defection, or to give any assistance to rugby league, a code that had raped the once-amateur game of its best talent for over a hundred years. Nor were the French courts interested in issuing an injunction order that would order him back to Belmore and thus prevent him playing for Toulon.

The bosses of the English Premier League aren't about to block all that foreign capital coming into the sport. They point out that their two most successful and best-run clubs, Manchester United and Chelsea, are owned by foreigners—America's Glazer family and Russia's Roman Abramovich respectively. Yet these two clubs, along with Liverpool and Arsenal—the fabled Big Four of the EPL—are responsible for about a third of the EPL's $8 billion debt. So what happens if this debt is called in, or foreign capital dries up, or the owners of clubs (including the owners of the NRL's Rabbitohs and Sea Eagles) tire of propping up the balance sheet?

The bottom line with privately owned clubs linked to international finance was exposed with the Global Financial Crisis. Man U's naming rights sponsor, an American insurance company, had to be bailed out by the US Government, so American taxpayers ended up underwriting an English team for $100 million. The owner of West Ham, Iceland's Bjorgolfur Gudmundsson, owned his country's second-biggest bank and saw it taken over by the government; he responded by asking £250 million for West Ham, despite paying £85 million a little over two years earlier.

I was back in England a year after the Storm trip and witnessed the reaction of EPL clubs to the GFC. Hicks had sent a messenger to speak to one of Kuwait's richest families about a sale and Abramovich, the Russian Croesus, had ordered his players to pay for their own training ground meals. But eight months later, Abramovich was back in the money, taking possession of a yacht with 25 suites, two swimming pools, a missile launcher and an anti-paparazzi shield—the shield fired lasers at digital cameras, destroying their pictures. And a Russian mining and media magnate, Alisher Usmanov, was locked in an old-fashioned cold war with American sports owner, Stan Kroenke, for control of Arsenal.

The problem is not the nationalities of these new owners (or, closer to home, the 'blow-in' reputations of NRL club co-owners), it's their durability. Usmanov's interest in the Gunners is said to be inspired by one of Abramovich's motives in owning Chelsea—acquiring a stake in a high-profile foreign club helps to protect other assets at home from official prying. Liverpool supporters are certainly entitled to ask if their owners love the club, or view it merely as a loss leader on a global balance sheet.

Bulldog officials and Liverpool fans might rail about wealthy overseas owners buying/selling the family silver, but sport is powerless to prevent globalisation. Even the Australian Football League, the second most successful national competition of an indigenous sport in the world (only America's NFL is more successful) is reaching out, staging matches in Dubai, London, and Shanghai running coaching programs in South Africa and paying for a full-time development officer in China.

For years it was assumed the AFL's uniqueness guaranteed its success—it was quarantined from other sports and countries because its players couldn't be poached by foreign codes. But when some of its top-punt kickers, recruited by NFL clubs in the United States, began reaching the 2009 Super Bowl at a time when TV rights fees in Australia had plateaued, the AFL began spending money overseas and recruiting from other sports. It poached one of rugby league's biggest stars, Karmichael Hunt, who had been born in Auckland to a Cook Island mother and a Samoan father, to play for its new Gold Coast team. The AFL didn't pay Hunt $700,000 a season because of his kicking and tackling skills, but to send a message—come and play our game—to Polynesian youngsters living in Queensland and western Sydney, where it was also setting up a franchise. The AFL's desperation to sign Hunt extended to them allowing him to play the 2009 off season with French rugby union club, Biarritz, rather than learn his new game. Should Hunt eventually debut with Gold Coast when the team enters the 2011 AFL competition, he will have became the first footballer to play in the elite league of three codes.

Hunt's signing was followed in June 2010 by the announcement the AFL's new Western Sydney team had signed the Brisbane Broncos' Israel Folau on a deal worth $6 million over four years. Folau, with spring-loaded feet and hands the size of oven mitts, is very skilled at catching the high ball. More significantly, his Tongan parentage is another enticement to the Polynesian Youth of New South Wales and Queensland to come and play AFL. His signing was proclaimed in the middle of the NRL's State of Origin series, raining on rugby league's parade and extracting further promotion for the AFL's invasion into the northern states.

'The most globalised business in the world, and the most lucrative, is the drug trade', says prominent political historian Walter LaFeber, author of *Michael Jordan and the New Global Capitalism*. 'But for legitimate businesses, sports is probably No. 1.' Globalisation is the mantra of the big football and basketball clubs and Formula I teams, using their celebrities to flog merchandise. Even individual athletes are now thinking globally.

US basketballer LeBron James, of the Cleveland Cavaliers, boasts his aim is to become a global sporting phenomenon, taking equity in companies that use his image rather than being paid straight sponsorship fees. With 37 tattoos including 'Gifted child' on his chest and 'Chosen 1' on his back, he admits his favourite line from the *Godfather* movie is 'Move while you have the muscle'. The fan clubs of Federer, or Beckham or Woods respect no borders: cults of every kind establish their homes everywhere. Even the few indifferent to sport are surrounded by the personalities and by the stunning advertising campaigns to promote them. We are titillated by the cult of celebrity—even by the criminal trials of past and present sportsmen, such as O.J. Simpson and another basketballer, Kobe Bryant.

The Super Bowl is the annual Sabbath of the American religion, the intersection of sport and commerce, the only time half the nation's population watches both the football and the commercials. Companies willingly pay US$3 million for a 30-second spot. At most points on a map, there are kids in Nike shoes, wearing NBA caps, drinking Gatorade and desperate to be of an age where they can enter the ubiquitously placed sports bars thoughout the world. All to watch a veritable Videohenge of sport on banks of TV screens. Enter these cavernous multistoreyed Shangri-las and you quickly understand the word 'fan' derives from the word 'fanatic'. TVs of all kinds hum, with some fans locked in private booths watching the action on minature, personal sets.

These palaces, where few words are exchanged, evoke thoughts in some writers of Kubrickian fantasies. Developments in technology will allow some wealthy fans to have their own home studios, further diminishing the contact between followers of a tribe. The allegiance of these fans to the NBA, or NFL, or EPL, is likely to come at the expense of a local team, an indigenous sport or a native cultural touchstone. Heard the one about the Eskimo on an ice floe who, when finally rescued, asks, 'How did Man U go against Chelsea?'

In some ways the rope ladder to the rescue helicopter is a metaphor for sport and globalisation, as clubs frantically climb to larger media markets. And Man United? If only. Rather than sport uniting man, Manchester United can be accused of exploiting man. Arguably the most famous sporting club in the world, its major shareholder, a Florida-based billionaire with interests in other American sporting franchises, is more interested in selling red shirts to Red China than spreading the gospel of the game. On the other hand, their supporters already believe they have conquered the globe, chanting, 'Ob-la-di, ob-la-da, Man United, champion of Planet Earth'. Like the New York Yankees, Man U is the globally marketable uberteam that every sport covets.

Sport has infected our accounting of nearly everything, and soccer, the world game, is the best at chasing sporting profit across borders. International sport dates back to the nineteenth century and the financial exploitation of sport is even older, but what is new is the degree of commercialisation and its spread to emerging markets. This was the thinking behind the English Premier League's aborted plan to add an 'international round' to its 38-game schedule—a round of matches played offshore, but mainly in Asian, African and Middle Eastern cities.

The idea for this '39th step' was to play ten fixtures in five different cities across the world in the middle of a two-week break in the domestic English season every January. The early reaction of Sepp Blatter, the boss of soccer's international body FIFA, was to say, 'I don't really know whether I should be appalled or whether I should laugh about it'. The plan was ultimately aborted, possibly because opposition from Asia and Africa may have jeopordised England's bid to stage the 2018 FIFA World Cup.

A rising-tide-lifts-all-boats argument was used to justify the EPL's plans, with English club bosses arguing a Man U versus Chelsea game in Shanghai would lift interest in soccer in the world's biggest country, China. Bollocks, as the English would say. It's merchandising and sponsorship opportunities—most importantly, additional TV broadcasting revenue—they seek.

According to Deloitte, the accounting firm that publishes an annual review of soccer's finances, most of the increase in the revenue of the 'big five' European leagues comes from broadcasting, bringing in at least 35 per cent of the total. Furthermore, foreign TV now accounts for a quarter of the EPL's broadcasting revenue, up from ten per cent only six years earlier. This was a major selling point used by the proponents of the 39th step to the EPL clubs because, unlike domestic TV revenues, foreign fees are shared evenly among clubs.

If broadcasting is a club's main source of revenue and the international yield is rising and is shared equally, why not? For that matter, it might even up a lopsided league in which the top-four clubs share the trophies. But fans don't think this way, as their reaction to the international round showed. They cherish the symmetry of their twenty team football league, where every team plays each other twice—once at home and once away. An additional round might be a gift win for Man U if it was drawn against, say, Stoke City.

Fans are fickle beasts and Manchester City fans, forever living in the shadow of the their more famous cousin, didn't object to the globalisation plans of their former chairman, Thaksin Shinawatra, the deposed prime minister of Thailand. He boasted, during my brief visit with the Storm, that he wanted to transform Manchester City and develop a network of the club's training and recruitment academies across Asia. 'There will be Man City China, Man City Japan, Man City US,' he said. 'In the next season, Man City will be another Man United.'

With £800 million of his assets frozen after the Thai coup in September 2006, club supporters hoped some of these assets, if released, would mean he would ratchet up his financial commitment to the club. After all, with a personal wealth put at £1.5 billion, it offered some hope Man City could match the Man U juggernaut. But Shinawatra experienced some difficulty releasing his money from Thailand and ownership of the club passed to a syndicate of Abu Dhabi billionaires who handed the manager a fat cheque book to buy up players and placate the fans.

One of their first targets was Brazilian Kaká, the 2007 World Footballer of the Year, who played for Milan, owned by another former prime minister, Italy's Silvio Berlusconi, a politician who has also been the focus of corruption and sex scandals. The reported transfer fee they offered was a potential record-breaking deal of €105 million, equivalent to paying each player in Australia's A-League $1million a year for two years. Kakà rejected Manchester City's offer of half-a-million pounds a week to stay with Milan, where he was earning €9 million a season, prompting the mealy-mouthed Berlusconi to say, 'He has higher values.'

But in June 2009, transfer fees and footballer salaries broke through the stratosphere. AC Milan succumbed to an offer from Spanish club Real Madrid, who paid £56 million for Kaká. Four days later, Manchester United's Cristiano Ronaldo became the most expensive footballer in history when Real Madrid agreed to pay to Man U an £80 million transfer fee and indulge the Portuguese peacock with more than £100 million in wages over the six-year duration of his contract. Six months earlier, Man U manager Sir Alex Ferguson had said, 'Do you think I would enter into a contract with that mob? I would not sell them a virus.'

While most English soccer clubs have been bought for the money they generate—media rights, ticket sales and merchandising—a couple are rich men's toys. Fulham is owned by Harrods' proprietor, Al Fayed, the father of Dodi, killed in the Parisian car chase with Princess Diana; Flavio Briatore, the playboy Italian, co-owns Queens Park Rangers, which plays in the tier below Premier League. Briatore's partners are Bernie Ecclestone and Lakshmi Mittal, an Indian iron and steel magnate, one of the world's richest men, who owns fifteen per cent of the club.

Ecclestone is a perfect go-to man for the EPL bosses and their globalisation plans. Over the years he has made some grandiose claims in the name of globalisation. Formula 1 advertising claims its races are watched by 54 billion people a year—a cumulative audience figure which could also be taken to mean every man, woman and child watches nine races a year. F1 racing has been relentlessly stretching from its old haunts in western Europe, the Americas and Japan towards the oil-rich Middle East and Asia's booming economies. A Malaysian Grand Prix was added in 1999; races have been held in Bahrain and China since 2004, Turkey since 2005 and the first night race was held in Singapore in 2008. Bernie's mate at QPR, Mittal, has been instrumental in India having a race in 2010. 'We go where the markets for the manufacturers are, where they are going to sell their cars in the future', Ecclestone has been quoted as saying.

That's bad news for Australia with its population of 22 million. But Ecclestone had already threatened Melbourne with the loss of its Grand Prix unless it moved to a later starting time in order to reach more overseas TV sets in more viewer-friendly hours. 'It is ridiculous that people are asked not to sleep in order to see it live', he said, clearly conveying the view Australians aren't people but props. The Victorian Government, forced to find a compromise between the evening start demanded by Ecclestone and a daytime race, opted for a twilight start. Despite losing financially on the race, the Victorians said the 'economic benefit' justified the changed time.

The volatile Australian dollar also renders the country vulnerable to the loss of many of its international sporting events, although the oft-quoted 'tyranny of distance', our 'out-of-sync' time zone and relatively small market play a role. But the rise of competing sporting venues, particularly in the Middle East and Asia, will be a major challenge, most notably for the Australian Open tennis tournament, one of four Grand Slam contests on the traditional calendar. For this reason, its organisers have taken deliberate steps to embrace Asia and the Pacific, to the extent of importing ball boys and girls from Korea, India and Singapore, and allocating places to two wild cards from Asia. The prospect of a Dubai, Chennai or Shanghai Open displacing the Australian Open in the Grand Slam tournament is a genuine fear, with the president of the Asian Tennis Federation, Anil Khanna, saying during the 2008 tournament, 'The aspiration of the people is there, the money power is there, the desire to do so is there in a number of countries in Asia, not just one'.

It's not as if Asia doesn't have its own top players competing in the Australian Open, compared to the host country where results from home-grown players over the past decade have been disappointing. Still, organisers have worked fervently to 'Asianise' the Australian Open, seeking a sponsorship with a Korean motoring manufacturer to replace the locally made Ford, and linking with three Asian broadcasters. The Open has changed radically from the tournament played 21 years earlier at Kooyong in Melbourne's affluent southeastern suburbs, where ball boys from local private schools attended to the players. This was an era when obscure Americans, rather than world No. 1s, won the event. Radio journalists were required to clean their booths of the deceased pidgeons that had accumulated there over the previous twelve months. Two decades later, those booths were replaced by state-of-the-art TV studios beaming matches into Asia.

Just as sport's capital markets are becoming more global and the developing economies—principally India with cricket—are creating their own product markets, there is also an increasing international integration of sport's labour markets. With seven languages spoken in the players' lounge at Man U, the big Red

Machine could be called Man United Nations. Kaká is one of many top footballers from Brazil playing in the rich European leagues, and that South American country is also a huge exporter of talent to developing leagues. Most clubs in the Asian Champions League boast at least one player from Brazil. The Brazilian known simply as Fred, as well as another two of his countrymen, delivered Melbourne Victory their first premiership in Football Federation Australia's fledgling A-League.

The supply side of soccer's labour market is finally catching up with the demand, which first announced itself 30 years ago when Tottenham Hotspurs shocked England by signing up two members of Argentina's World Cup winning team. Imports into Europe are now so commonplace that both FIFA and its European confederation, UEFA, would like to impose a cap on numbers but European Union labour laws allow players to move freely between member states. The EPL is tackling the issue of shrinking home-grown talent by enforcing a quota system next season, where eight of a team's squad of 25 must have been registered with the club for three years prior to turning 21. The new rule is designed to ultimately strengthen the English national team. However, some of the EPL's top coaches, such as Arsenal's Arsene Wenger and Liverpool's Rafael Benitez, reject such cultural protectionism as counterproductive and myopic.

The most-talented players will always want to gravitate towards the wealthiest employers, whose capacity to pay is further enhanced by the rich TV contracts these brilliant superstars generate. Because England has the richest TV contracts in soccer, more than half the players in the EPL are from outside the United Kingdom, up from one quarter ten years earlier. The concentration of players in English soccer produced a bizarre scenario at

Euro 2008: one eighth of the players in the tournament came from English clubs, yet the national team failed to qualify.

This was one of the reasons Italy and Spain banned foreigners in the early 1960s, after nearly two decades of vigorously recruiting top overseas players. At that time, fervent nationalism arrested the power of globalisation but not for long. Spain lifted its ban in 1974 and Italy followed in 1980: both of them opting for club over country and conceding the riches of a cosmopolitan club competition overrule the importance of providing the environment for the development of a national team.

The hollowness of soccer's hectoring boast to other sports that it is the world game is exposed by the concentration of talent in about a dozen big clubs in six countries. England's top-four clubs, Scotland's Glasgow Celtic and Rangers, Holland's PSV and Ajax, Germany's Bayern Munich, Spain's Real Madrid and Barcelona, Italy's AC Milan and Juventus and France's Olympique Lyonnais dominate domestic competitions. Soccer may well be played all over the globe but in terms of winning, it's a game for twelve European cities.

America's game, baseball, has also undergone internationalisation of talent. Ten years ago, the proportion of players in the major leagues born outside the United States was twenty per cent; now it is 30 per cent. Most are from Central America, with Dominicans having the biggest representation, although Japanese and Taiwanese are also making an impact. In the minor leagues, the proportion is higher.

Nigeria is the go-to place for the top agents of America's National Basketball Association, who are investing more time and money in more places searching for precious resources—in other words, seven footers. The No. 1 draft choice in 2008 in the

NBA was Australia's Andrew Bogut, a $76 million man. The tallest player in the NBA, and one of the best, is the Houston Rockets' Yao Ming of China.

Similarly, over 30 per cent of players in the US National Hockey League emanate from outside North America, with Scandinavians and Russians popular. Over 30 Samoans play in the the US National Football League. Polynesians are also attracted to the physical nature of the two rugby codes: one quarter of players in the NRL are sons of the South Pacific, while the proportion in the feeder leagues is approaching 50 per cent. Tongans, Samoans, Fijians and New Zealand Maoris are also heavily represented in Australian and Kiwi Super Rugby teams.

Africa has become a significant source of soccer talent in recent years, exposing the shameful side of globalisation. Young African kids, wearing the faded and torn strips of teams from across Europe, are scouted playing on beaches and in townships and herded into football schools, with hypocritical biblical names, such as 'Sons of Moses' and 'Lovers of Christ'. Children have become the object of a transaction, deceived by a distant dream and denied the opportunity of an education and the joy of growing up in a loving family. Unlicensed agents recruit skinny Ghanaian kids as young as ten, convincing their gullible parents to part with the cost of a sea passage to Europe, where they are trafficked into youth teams in Belgian, French and Dutch cities. If the player fails to earn a contract, he is abandoned as yet another black illegal immigrant in Europe.

Ten years ago, about half the players at the African national championships played in their own countries, with about 40 per cent with European clubs. But now, the differential has been reversed, with more than a half playing in Europe and less than one-third at home in domestic leagues, mainly in north Africa.

Ironically, young Australian cricketers may find themselves abandoned in their own country because of the popularity of cricket in India—a vivid manifestation of the shift in this global sport's economy from the wealthy countries to the developing economies. The spectacular, almost overnight, success of the Indian Premier League has shaken cricket from the bottom to the top. The attraction of the IPL lies in its format: Twenty20 cricket is an abbreviated form of the game, where each team bowls twenty overs and matches last about three hours. It appeals to the instant-gratification, no-dead-air generation, where they must always have something to amuse, and to a TV audience, offering a night's entertainment with powerful shots to the boundaries and beyond. The term 'crickertainment' was coined to reflect the IPL's interest in entertaining the crowd, rather than in the contest itself.

As a further irony, Twenty20 was invented in England as a means of attracting a different demographic to those who traditionally watched county cricket. The Board of Control for Cricket in India initially opposed it but, when their team beat Pakistan in the final of the inaugural World Twenty20 Cup held in South Africa, the new game was an instant hit in a country where cricket is 30 to 40 times more popular than the next most-watched sport. While the stepping stones on the IPL path are paved in gold, they may yet prove to be tombstones for some young Australians. This was evident when New South Wales chose the big-hitting New Zealander, Brendon McCullum, in their team for the domestic Twenty20 final against Victoria, even though the Blues had already qualified for the Champions League tournament in India in October 2009, where the best two teams from each of the main cricketing nations would compete for a first prize of US$3 million.

The justification for depriving a NSW player a place in the Blues' final team was that McCullum needed to qualify for the team going to India and Cricket NSW feared some of their regular players would not be available for the tournament, owing to their contractual commitments to IPL teams for whom they had played earlier in the year. Previously, McCullum could only have qualified for the tournament if his IPL team, the Kolkata Knight Riders, had been one of India's two top teams, but it wasn't. It meant that the big-bashing Kiwi played Twenty20 cricket in 2009 for teams from three nations—New Zealand, Australia and India—while a young NSW player, who may have played all season and helped the Blues reach the final, missed out.

Cricket Australia did not raise any objections; Victoria, which lost the Twenty20 final to New South Wales on the last ball, merely expressed disappointment they hadn't thought of drafting the Kiwi first. Initially, Cricket Australia's worst fears about India's highly compressed Twenty20 season was that its Test players might retire early, to capitalise on contracts where they receive more money for six weeks' work in India than they earn for the rest of the year. Or that young Australians at the base of the playing pyramid might opt for IPL's riches rather than endure the long apprenticeship before they win their first baggy green cap. Ultimately, the Blues won the Champions League tournament without McCullum playing, but the episode showed the riches of Twenty20 cricket in India had more widespread impact than anyone imagined.

*

The argument in favour of awarding places in domestic teams to foreign imports has traditionally been that this is a fair trade-off for the billions of dollars the sport will earn in international revenue. It's a fair argument when the US NBA games featuring Yao Ming are being sold to a nation with 1.3 billion people, but it doesn't stack up with India and cricket. India generates 70 per cent of the world's cricket revenue, meaning international sales of the IPL are insignificant, compared to earnings from TV within the country. So, for every Indian player replaced by a young Australian, the overseas earnings are paltry.

Foreign players do add interest inside India, though, as evidenced to me when, after a horrendous holiday riding a camel in Rajasthan, I happily walked though the crowded street of Jaipur and, looking up at the billboards, saw the smiling face of Australia's Brett Lee endorsing products. This was one year before the advent of the IPL—Lee had recorded a hit song with a Bollywood glamour actress as a foretaste of the exotic mix overseas stars now add to India's domestic game. The big money hires foreign superstars who win the championship and satisfy the fans. Furthermore, importing players sends a powerful message to the ICC of India's hold over the sport.

Given international cricket's TV revenue sharing agreement, Cricket Australia is not likely to object to the loss of its young players. After all, Australia earns four times more from India touring Australia than it does from a visit by any other country. When India tours Australia, as they will in 2011–12, Australia receives all the revenue and India is simply paid its expenses; the reverse applies when Australia tours India.

Australia's tacit acceptance of the IPL stands in stark contrast to the opposition Kerry Packer encountered when, having been rebuffed in his attempts to secure for his Nine Network the TV rights to cricket, he started his World Series Cricket revolution and embraced the new phenomenon, one-day cricket. It was called 'pyjama cricket' then, but now the 50-over game risks being overtaken by the even shorter version. Packer told the Australian Cricket Board when he finally got them to the table, 'There's a little bit of the whore in all of us, gentlemen. What's your price?'

India adopted the same mercenary course with the IPL, awarding teams to eight cities, rather than the 26 states. The franchises were auctioned to a heady mix of corporate moguls and film stars, linking business and Bollywood glamour. Scarcity created value and bidded up the price of the teams, whose names included Royals and Kings but could all just as easily be called Sacred Cash Cows. Slickly packaged, it's a telegenic property with charismatic stars; it's sport as entertainment, while also occupying a significant place on the Indian cultural vanguard. With scantily clad cheerleaders, noisy bands, fireworks, even spectators watching in spas, the closing ceremony to the season featured a cast of superstars in a Bollywood dancing spectacular.

Although the IPL owners are capitalist, the league is socialist. Spending on players is capped and franchises share TV revenue and central sponsorship. One of News Corporation's likely heirs, Lachlan Murdoch, invested modestly in the cheapest franchise, the Jaipur-based Rajasthan Royals, which won the final of the inaugural competition on the last ball of the match. Australia's Shane Warne, captain–coach of the Royals, assessed the interest generated to be greater than anything he had ever experienced, including Ashes series. Significantly, the final was played in front of a TV audience of hundreds of millions, at the same time as the Australian Test team was playing before an audience of a few thousand in the West Indies.

The second IPL final, won by Adam Gilchrist's Deccan Chargers, featured two teams who were bottom of the ladder the previous year, suggesting the salary cap system certainly works. Or is it the sheer unpredictability of Twenty20? Zimbabwe can beat Australia; the Netherlands can defeat England. There is no pattern to its success, unlike Australia's long period of domination of test cricket. India won the first Twenty20 world championship; Pakistan the second and Trinidad and Tobago belted it out with New South Wales in the Champions League final. In any case, the IPL salary cap may not last for long. India is sheering away from its socialist past at industrial speed.

The second season was played in South Africa because of political turmoil in India. Crowds were down but moving an entire competition offshore demonstrated how global sport has become. As Makhaya Ntini, one of the IPL players, said, 'I am a black player, playing for a team in the south of India, getting paid in US dollars for playing in the Indian Premier League in South Africa.' It evoked memories of another event which attracted global attention: an English princess and an Arab merchant prince travelling in a German car chased by Italian photographers, crashing in a French tunnel . . . you get the idea.

Is the IPL an example of 'globalisation' or, as writer Gideon Haigh terms it, 'Indianisation'? The second IPL season demonstrated the imposition of Indian commercial and cultural values on cricket. IPL commissioner Lalit Modi sounded as if he was the boss of an Imperial Premier League when he spoke of the benefits to South Africa via the airfares and hotel expenses incurred. In fact, as a means of keeping it outside the ICC's jurisdiction, the

BCCI argue the IPL and Champions League are not global tournaments but domestic competitions.

Lalit's modi operandi is the entertainment of the Indian cricket fan. Game times are determined by the availability of domestic TV time slots—arrangements to suit what has been called 'the lanyard wearing classes'. The second IPL season was a satellite India on South African soil. But Modi's innings came to an end at the conclusion of the third IPL season, when he stood up at the presentation ceremony to the winners, the Chennai Super Kings, and acknowledged accusations of lack of transparency in the league. The BCCI, which owns the IPL, suspended him immediately after his valedictory speech. A compulsive Twitterer, he had revealed that an investor in one of the IPL's new teams was a girlfriend of India's deputy foregin minister. The woman had been given her substantial stake in the team for free. The minister was forced to resign but Congress retaliated by unleashing a tax audit of the IPL's finances. The money pouring into cricket and the glamour lured the politicians but the type of scrutiny the buccaneering Modi was attracting was not part of the plan.

Nevertheless, marketing dollars will still follow the success of the IPL because sport is still the most effective vehicle for reaching males. India has over 350 TV channels; the fragmentation of audiences everywhere has given the most popular sports enormous bargaining power globally. In most countries, as the number of channels has multiplied, it has become harder to reach larger audiences through any single channel, but cricket in India has retained its ability to meet this need of advertisers. For advertisers in India forever in search of expanding their markets, cricket is king—whether the sales they seek are in Mumbai or a remote village in the Deccan.

The appeal of Twenty20 cricket to the instant-gratification, short attention-span generation is mirrored in changes in the media where the news is now delivered online. In fact, the three forms of cricket probably correspond to the three ways newspaper journalists present stories. We have the Test cricket pieces—the Saturday long reads where the work is carefully researched and written over a week, the shape of the story changing as more information comes to hand; the 50-over story, the one you see in your Monday to Friday newspaper—it tells the bare story but is at least 12 hours out of date by the time you read it; and online stories, like Twenty20 cricket, which are immediate, attention grabbing but also often inaccurate and occasionally risky.

Interestingly, other abbreviated forms of sport haven't taken off like Twenty20 cricket. Arena football, the ship-in-the-bottle form of NFL in the United States, failed. Rugby union enthusiasts prefer Test matches to the Sevens game of seven men-a-side and seven-minute halves. It's backseat lovemaking compared to a romantic dinner; it's a Reader's Digest condensed book version of *War and Peace*. Perhaps it will change now that the IOC have allowed Sevens Rugby into the Olympic temple. It will debut at the Rio de Janeiro Olympics of 2016, where the throw-the-ball-around style will complement the carnival atmosphere of the Games.

Perhaps the strongest consequence of globalisation is that it confers power to the dominant cultures. For years, political scientists have talked of the deployment of 'soft power'—a country's use of culture and information, such as films and fashion, music and consumer goods, to win over foreigners. The United States has certainly challenged this theory by deploying its military power in Iraq and Afghanistan but, essentially, 'soft power', transported in nanoseconds by the information technology revolution, has proved more effective than political bastardry or military brawn, or even trade sanctions, as a way of exerting influence.

I visited a Cuban sports institute prior to the Sydney Olympics and saw buses abandoned because the American-made spare parts needed to get them back on the road were unavailable as a result of the trade blockade. Yet athletes there were secretly listening to American music in their crowded dormitories. As Thomas Freidman writes in *The World is Flat*, the explosion of technology means that people are connected all over the planet, far more easily than ever before.

Sport is the new soft power and it's difficult to escape the notion cricket will grease the skids of India's push to sell its films and culture overseas. India's official national sport is field hockey, yet a former captain of the national team said, 'Everything is going for cricket. And nothing for hockey or any other sport in India. Everyone concentrates only on promoting cricket. Mileage, publicity, sponsorship. Name it and everything goes towards cricket, leaving barely half a per cent for the other sports.'

Could the day come where Indian cricket will be bigger in Australia than Australian cricket is in India? In other words, will there be more interest by Australians in IPL and matches played on the subcontinent than there is interest by Indians in an Australian touring team? The increasing number of expatriate Indians wanting to watch games from home could guarantee this. Cricket Australia's third-biggest revenue stream from the overseas sale of media rights—after India and the UK—comes from North America where cricket is a very minor game. Expatriate populations—principally Indians subscribing to cable TV—drive this. As a Cricket Australia spokesman says, 'Indian IT experts living in New York buy cricket bats for kids living in Alice Springs.' In other words, the cable TV subscriptions paid by the Indian IT experts in New York fund the rights income paid to Cricket Australia, which uses some of the money to buy equipment for disadvantaged Australian youth.

Even Warne, who a decade earlier had tins of baked beans airfreighted to the Australian team's Chennai hotel because he didn't like the local tucker, pleaded with the International Cricket Council to quarantine a place for the IPL in the sport's ever-expanding calendar. His motive was clear: the stars of the game should not be forced to choose between club and country; that is, deciding between representing IPL clubs in the annual tournament or playing for their national team in matches elsewhere.

Xenophobia, once blatant in most sports, is diminishing rapidly. NASCAR's Jimmy Spencer once lamented Toyota's presence in the truck-racing series because the Japanese 'bombed Pearl Harbor, after all', and LPGA golfer Jan Stephenson whined that 'the Asians are killing our tour'. Such comments would attract massive fines and apologies today. As the world seemingly grows simultaneously smaller and more complex, sport is the connective tissue.

Globalisation is like sport: for all the winners, there are, necessarily, losers as well. Soccer and basketball chiefs evangelise that their worldwide sprawl is a blessing to leagues in other nations using that rising-tide-lifts-all-boats argument to justify their global push. But it doesn't always work out that way: some boats run aground. With globalisation, peril rides tandem with promise. American football's European league, set up in the 1990s, has been abandoned, principally because there was no interest in a second-rate competition. If you're an American living in Europe, why pay to watch the London Monarchs play when you can stay home and see decidedly superior NFL games on TV?

Basketball in Australia is a fascinating case. In the late 1980s and early 1990s, it rode the wave of the world-wide boom caused partly by the Jordan phenomenon and clever NBA marketing. Fans watched NBA games on TV and this may have even stimulated interest in the local product. Nor was the loss of some great local players—such as Luc Longley, Andrew Gaze, Chris Anstey and Shane Heal—to overseas leagues seen as a negative. But by the mid 1990s, basketball chiefs in Australia sensed the game was treading water and switched to a summer schedule in order not to compete with AFL and the rugby codes. Media magnates Kerry Stokes (owner of Channel Seven) and Rupert Murdoch (owner of the Brisbane Bullets team) agitated hardest for the change. However, the less wealthy private owners of some of the NBL clubs did not devote sufficient funds to making the league work and player payments persistently put team finances under pressure.

The Sydney Kings for a time were the exception, but the team began losing in the 1990s and its fickle fans tired of a mediocre, if profitable, team. The TV networks were not interested in a league without a strong Sydney team and when Kings' owner Mike Wrublewski took his team to the Homebush Olympic precinct, crowds declined even further. After Wrublewski there was a succession of owners, as there were with the Brisbane Bullets. Firepower, the company that claimed to have invented a petrol pill, sponsored the Kings and Eddy Groves, the owner of the ABC Learning childcare chain, backed the Bullets. But the finances of both sponsors collapsed spectacularly. When the new eight-team competition began in September 2009, the Sydney Kings, once involved in one of the most-thrilling final series seen, had died. It took some time before there was any business interest in resuscitating them and they are set to enter the 2010 competition. But the European leagues—Italy, Greece, Croatia and Russia—have also retreated from the heady days of the 1990s when 'His Airness', Michael Jordan, ruled the courts.

While globalisation may be blamed for the decline of basketball in Australia, it's probably more accurate to accuse private ownership. Australia could not attract long-term owners of clubs and the sport momentarily leapt up higher than its natural place in the pecking order, only to sink back where it belonged. But it will never die on TV.

Sport is the world's largest supplier of reality programming and the explosion of broadband and the proliferation of TV tiers has created the so-called 'thousand channel universe'. This universe may end up being a blessing for niche sports. In the same way your local newsagency seems to have a magazine on even the most obscure topics, there will be a TV platform for every sport.

TV has led to the 'Balkanisation' of some sports. The alphabet soup of sanctioning bodies in world boxing, together with a subdivision of weight classes, means the WBO's (World Boxing Organisation) light-welterweight bouts are seen on some obscure cable network, or ethnically targetted pay-for-view. In fact, what was once sport's most glamorous property—the heavyweight championship of the world—has had four simultaneous champions.

Compare this with the story told after Jack Dempsey scythed down Jess Willard to win the world heavyweight title on American Independence Day 1919, a bout won under a blazing hot sun in Toledo. Dempsey later fell asleep in his hotel room and when he awoke, uncertain whether he had been dreaming, raced out onto the footpath to confront a passing paperboy who was selling extra editions of the *Toledo Blade*, which contained a report of the fight. 'Who's the heavyweight champion?' Dempsey asked desperately, according to a *Sports Illustrated* report years later. The boy gaped at him and answered, 'You are, you dope!'

What is the most anachronistic aspect of this story? Bouts fought at midday? Paperboys? Extra editions in the age of online? The use of the word 'dope'? Or is it that a kid today would not recognise a world champion, unless it was, say, Mike Tyson? Today, we're more likely to see a 'Thriller in Vanilla' than Ali versus Frazier.

For every sporting team trying to extend its market, there is a countervailing trend to stop it becoming too big for its boots, particularly its football boots. AFL team, North Melbourne, changed its name to the Kangaroos, hoping to widen its appeal past its base in the inner west of Melbourne and seeking to be recognised across all of Australia. It didn't matter there was already another national team of Kangaroos—the Australian rugby league team. The experiment failed and the Kangaroos finally decided their home was Arden Street, north Melbourne, even though they lived out of old containers until their new clubhouse was built. North, as they are also known, rejected an AFL bid for them to relocate north, to the Gold Coast; settled with their shareholder owners; reverted to the membership model of other Melbourne clubs; and became North Melbourne again.

Similarly, NRL team, the Cronulla Sutherland Sharks, who had once thought they could widen their market with a non-geographical name and called themselves Sharks, eventually concluded their home was Cronulla. They survive in territory wholly surrounded by the St George Illawarra Dragons, a team that merged from the territories north and south of Cronulla. In any case, any thought they had a monopoly on 'sharks' is overcome by a Sharks team in South Africa playing in Super Rugby.

Rugby union's attempt to name its teams Hurricanes, Crusaders, Bulls and Stormers, without any reference to geography, has failed—most Australians don't know whether these teams are from New Zealand or South Africa. Nor did the name Super 14 make it clear that it referred to 14 teams. When this competition was initially launched, in the early 1990s as Super 12, adman John Singleton, a rugby union fan and a marketing genius, thought it meant there would be twelve (instead of the usual fifteen) players on the field. Nor is Super Rugby expanding the sport's market—games are shown on pay TV, rather than free-to-air, and often after midnight.

Some sports will continue to delude themselves they are a global game. When an American National Football League (NFL) team wins the Super Bowl, it calls itself 'world champion', despite the 32 competing teams all being based in the United States. British funnyman John Cleese has a very effective retort to this. Listing the reasons why Great Britain is superior to the United States, he says, 'When we hold a world championship for a particular sport, we invite teams from other countries'.

The Olympics, on the other hand, is for everyone. Except those who have opted to use sport as a protest, as the African nations did in 1976 (Montreal) in opposition to the presence of the apartheid-backed South African team. The United States and some of its allies boycotted the Moscow Games in 1980 as a protest against the Soviet Union's war in Afghanistan. The Soviet bloc retaliated four years later, sitting out the Los Angeles Olympics. Since then, the International Olympic Committee has been largely spared boycotts; however, from time to time it has pompously called upon warring nations in the Baltic States and Middle East to lay down their arms in order to allow some frolic in the snow, such as the Winter Olympics, to proceed in an environment of global peace. Nobody at the United Nations takes the IOC as seriously as it perceives itself, intent on its self-appointed role as intergalactic policeman. Still, 2500 years ago at the ancient Olympics, the Greek city states of Athens and Sparta would call a halt to their hostilities and maybe these modern-day ostriches at IOC headquarters in Lausanne really believe nations should do likewise, in order for the syncronised swimming to begin.

The IOC did bring China closer to the rest of the world via the Beijing Olympics—the coming out party of the world's largest nation—despite tensions between the Communist Government's intention to block some websites and the IOC's promise to journalists that there would be no censorship. A bizarre pre-Games experiment by the Chinese Government demonstrated their then anxiety about the media's attitude to protests over their occupation of Tibet. The Beijing Organising Committee invited a number of journalists to a big party, where free grog flowed and tables groaned with delicious food. Four hours into the soirée, with secret cameras filming from multiple angles, 'protestors' carrying a Tibetan flag burst into the room. The journalists merely chuckled and looked around for the waiter carrying the drinks. No-one reached for their notebooks. This staged protest taught the organisers nothing, except that journalists resemble footballers in their avidity to elbow their way past others to reach the spicy meatballs.

Almost all the world's nations turned up to Beijing, as well as the big corporations, demonstrating once again that the Olympics is a festival of global sport and business. It's a huge compliment to the Olympics, considering the athletes receive no prize money and sponsors are not permitted to advertise in the arenas. Nor is the IOC a profit-making body. Still, as Australia's Steven Bradbury discovered in 2002 when all the other short-track speed skaters in his race at Salt Lake City fell, win a gold medal and the financial rewards will follow.

For global companies, the games are a golden marketing opportunity. Summer and Winter Olympics were held in the same year until 1992 (in Barcelona, Spain, and Albertville, France) when it was decided to stage them two years apart (starting with Lillehammer in 1994 and Atlanta in 1996). The IOC marketing team reasoned that sponsorship demands were too heavily concentrated in one year and more marketing dollars could be earned if spread over a quadrennium.

For broadcasters, more eyeballs mean more advertisers and more pay TV subscribers. The broadcasting rights from Europe and the United States for the 2016 Summer Olympics were sold before the host city (Rio de Janeiro) was awarded. The Olympics are not the richest TV rights of all, sitting below FIFA's World Cup, but if the IOC aimed to maximise revenue, rather than reach, it could earn more. From that point of view, the IOC should also be lauded—delivering the Games to viewers in undeveloped countries and distributing its wealth via 'solidarity' programs in poor nations. It can lay more genuine claims to uniting man than, say Man United.

Furthermore, over a hundred years ago it invented the idea of foreign cities funding its operations. Every four years it finds another city to pay its bills, well before Manchester United and the other EPL teams cottoned on to the 'international round' idea, or Ecclestone pitted one Formula I bidding city against another.

Sonny Bill—nicknamed 'Money Bill' by Bulldogs supporters—did not play much football in his first season for Toulon. He spent most of the time sidelined with injury, while club owner Mourad Boudjellal, an eccentric businessman who earned his wealth from publishing comics, expressed anger his foreign legion of players did not cement the club in France's top division of fourteen clubs. While some suspect Sonny Bill's problems with injury, rather than his desire to eventually play for the All Blacks, was the main motivation for him switching codes and countries, there are other factors in the global spread of talent.

Money isn't always the main lure for leaguies to play rugby in France, although Europe's liberal tax laws are an incentive. NRL players may see it as a way to avoid the drudgery of full-time training, where they are breathalysed, weighed, tested for body fat and forced to endure hours of weights, tedious training drills and video replays. Many tire of the incessant media scrutiny and the questioning by club supporters on the relatively new fan forum of the internet. Switching to a less physically intense game is another reason, together with the desire for a more relaxed lifestyle at the end of a brutal career.

European-based agents talk up a world where players jet mid week to ski in the French Alps. Penrith's former NRL star Craig Gower joined Bayonne, a French rugby club, where he flew to Morocco to play golf. 'It's nicer than downtown Manchester', admits Gower's long-term manager, Greg Willett. Gower, who holds an Italian passport, was desperate to escape Sydney after highly publicised drunken behaviour on a Sunshine Coast golf course and in a Kings Cross bar. 'The French clubs rest the stars when they are playing a low side, allowing the top ones like Craig to spend the weekend staying at the Aman Hotel, Morocco,' says Willett. 'He's close to a group of Australian surfers who are based on France's Atlantic coast.' Gower has subsequently been chosen to represent Italy and now plays for an Italian club.

An even brighter NRL star with a stellar name, Mark Gasnier, switched to French rugby ahead of Sonny Bill. But globalisation and the thousand channel universe means there is a downside for Sonny Bill and Gasnier: they can no longer hide if they play a bad game. Thirty years ago American baseball star Reggie Jackson quipped with a degree of self-comforting indifference, 'When we lose and I strike out, a billion people in China don't care.' Well, today, quite a few of them do and they pay plenty of yuan to watch Americans play baseball at the Beijing Olympics.

Forty-five years ago, players from Sydney's Western Suburbs rugby league club travelled south on an ocean liner for the Melbourne Cup carnival, an extravagant end-of-season trip in those days. Maybe it was the broken noses and cauliflower ears, but some VFL stars out at Flemington suspected the group was Sydney footballers. Told the code was rugby league, one asked quite innocently, 'Is there a player up there in Sydney with a French-sounding name?' He was referring of course to St George's Reg Gasnier, the uncle of Mark and one of the code's original four Immortals. Similarly, most of the Magpies had only heard of a VFL player with an Italian-sounding name, the legendary Ron Barassi.

Today, however, NRL players are awestruck at the feats of Hawthorn's Buddy Franklin, while AFL players admire the Broncos' soaring Israel Folau and the mercurial Storm fullback, Billy Slater. Team-of-the-Century halfback Andrew Johns once asked me about the AFL club Geelong's talented young Ablett brothers, particularly 22-year-old Nathan, who retired after winning the grand final. I told him that many young athletes who grow up on the Bellarine peninsula prefer to work as trademen, downing tools when the surf is up, rather than attend football training. Instead of drinking Gatorade after training, they'd prefer to cut into a carton of beer after a surf. 'Tell me about it', Joey said wistfully.

Meanwhile, Sonny Bill completed his second season in Toulon and visited Australia, playing for a Barbarians team against the Wallabies. If he stays four years with Toulon, he will be eligible to play for France, making it the fourth country he could represent—he has antecedents in Tonga, was born in New Zealand and lived in Sydney for seven years, as well as having a grandmother living in Australia, meaning he is also eligible for these three countries as well. But his old team, the Bulldogs, true to their culture, finally came to the conclusion they didn't like this world outside the southwestern suburbs of Sydney. Back at the top of the NRL ladder, with a new team after cancelling the contracts of many of their Polynesian players, their board unanimously voted to call themselves the Canterbury Bankstown Bulldogs. (They had been known as the Berries between 1935 and 1977 when they decided to acquire a more aggressive name, choosing the bulldog mascot and becoming known as Canterbury, or the Bulldogs.) Then, in 1999, they became known simply as The Bulldogs. But in recognition of their strong Arab base in Bankstown and the attachment their supporters had to their retiring great Muslim point scorer, Hazem El Masri, the club changed its name officially to the Canterbury Bankstown Bulldogs.

And after a two-year break, Nathan Ablett decided to return to the AFL, signing with the new Gold Coast team on lucrative terms. The warmer water off Surfers Paradise would allow him to pursue his other passion, while taking him away from the Geelong spotlight where his father Gary and brother, Gary Jnr, are perhaps the best father–son combination in any sport at any time. Richer and more relaxed, Nathan now has the best of both worlds. Oh, and midway through 2010, Gasnier returned from France to play for St George Illawarra, while Sonny Bill, equally true to his roots, signed with a New Zealand club in order to represent the All Blacks at home in rugby's World Cup.

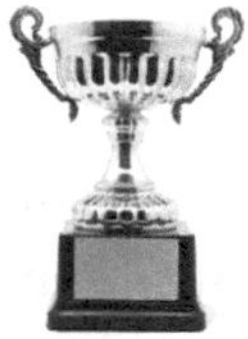

FOUR

SNEAKIER

It was a question I should never have asked a father in front of his son but the answer was worth the brief embarrassment. In October 1985, while 40 players from the three St George teams that played in the year's grand finals enjoyed themselves at Disneyland, California, I travelled to nearby Orange County to meet with Jack Kramer, the man who started world professional tennis. I'd often wondered whether those best of three-set matches in the early days of pro tennis were legitimate. After all, they rarely ended with the second set. The small crowds always seemed to get their money's worth. Did players like Pancho Gonzales and Lew Hoad agree to square the first two sets and play a fair dinkum decider?

In 1959–60, Kramer had seven players making over US$50,000 a year—more than the top US football and baseball players were earning. But there was little public acceptance of his players. The conservative, powerful administration of the amateur game dominated, running the major tennis tournaments at Wimbledon, Flushing Meadows and Roland Garros. The spin at the time was that if you were in favour of pro tennis, you were advocating the game be handed to Jack Kramer, a former US and Davis Cup champion. The nabobs who ran the

Grand Slam tournaments were obviously waiting for Kramer's circus to drown in a sea of red ink.

I wondered, as I attempted to play a game of golf with Kramer and his son, Ron, at Jack's country club in the hills of Orange County, did he fix matches to secure good gates? Golf games between Jack and Ron, a pro, were always tense, like the conflict in the *Kramer vs. Kramer* movie. Only a couple of strokes separated them on the last hole and the young pro was clearly sulky. But Jack muffed a putt to hand victory to his relieved son, and it seemed an appropriate time to raise the question of tennis fixes.

There was a long pause before Jack answered. I recall the shock on the face of the son at the hesitation and the possibility his father might have been involved in 'tanking', as it is called in the United States. 'No', Jack finally replied before adding, 'but there is one thing on my conscience—only one thing I regret in all my years of tennis. When I signed [Ken] Rosewall, I was afraid Gonzales would eat him alive. So I went to Gonzales and said, "If you find some way to carry the kid, it's worth another five per cent of the gross to you". But after the first four matches, Gonzales came to me and said, "I can't play when I'm thinking about trying to carry him". It was obvious that Gonzales was worried and it was also obvious that Rosewall wasn't the pushover any of us expected. I told Gonzales to forget the whole thing. You get screwed up when you try to lose.'

In other words, Kramer was messing with the paradox at the root of all sporting competition: to draw the most from a game, the athlete must play all-out to win while not allowing this obsession with victory to ruin the pleasure of his co-conspirator in the quest, his fellow competitor. Cheating is an outgrowth of obsession with winning, while game fixing is a perversion of competition (a word derived, significantly, from the Latin *com* and *petere*, 'to seek together').

Playing for pleasure—as opposed to playing for crowds, TV audiences, prize money and ATP points—was evident the night of a quarterfinal of the Australian Open in 1995 between two Americans, Jim Courier and Pete Sampras. Sampras had recently learned that his coach had brain cancer and was unlikely to live. Someone from the crowd at Melbourne Park called out with clumsy good intentions, 'Do it for your coach', and Sampras could not contain his emotions any longer and tears cascaded down his face. He was clearly experiencing difficulty sighting the ball on his serve and Courier cried out softly across the net, 'We don't have to do this, Pete'.

It's at times like this that sport can be compared to religion. All the world's major religions place a strong emphasis on charity, as is written in the bible (1 Corinthians 13:13): 'And now abideth faith, hope, charity, these three, but the greatest of these is charity.' It follows that the athlete should show his followers a generosity of spirit. Yet that charity has never been extended by the guardians of amateur games to those seeking to earn a living from their skills.

Kramer, who died in 2009, told me he had to make a sacrificial lamb of himself so that tennis could embrace professional players. 'In the end, in 1962, the fight had gone out of me', he said with a tinge of sadness. 'I tried everything and nothing ever worked. I had to leave or we'd never have seen an open game.' It took another six years before professionals and amateurs played together in Grand Slam tournaments. Tennis and golf for a long time resisted attempts to destroy their patina of purity and their status as bastions of the world's fast-fading amateurism. Traditionally, they had depended a great deal on the amateur ideal, which was not so much that athletes should be unpaid as that they were so privileged, by class and choice of games, that they had no need to be paid.

Tennis had a regal beginning as 'Royal Tennis', the game played by English kings, including Henry VIII. (It's not known whether the vigorous exercise at Hampton Court accelerated Henry's venereal disease which led to his death, or, as my late Catholic mother-in-law asserted, caused him to 'literally explode in his own filth'.) Modern tennis, as we know it, began when Major Walter Clopton Wingfield patented 'A Portable Court of Playing Tennis' on 23 February 1874. The following month, upper-class magazines, such as *The Court Journal*, *The Field* and the *Army and Navy Gazette* (catering for the British officer-class), reported the new game worldwide. It quickly spread to the south of France where English holidaymakers played it on the beaches. Wingfield, who called his game by the unwieldy name *Sphairistikè*, could not enforce his patent because it was a modification of an existing game. The patent expired on 23 February 1877, just before the first Wimbledon, an indication of the momentum the new game had gathered.

There are a number of reasons for its widespread success. An Englishman, Edwin Budding, invented the lawnmower and around this time the garden roller also emerged; these allowed croquet to be played on well-rolled, level courts with close-clipped grass. Croquet became the fad in the mid nineteenth century. And Charles Goodyear vulcanised rubber in 1860, leading to the bouncing ball. While Goodyear's name survives, he didn't profit from his invention. The Germans seized on the innovation and manufactured thin-walled balls—Major Wingfield's balls came from Germany.

Back then, golf clubs were called woods, because they were made of wood but sport's golden days of wood would soon be over. Change came via technological advances in other sports. Howard Head, an aircraft engineer who was a lousy skier, spent US$6000 he won in a poker game designing a metallic ski and the elite sport of alpine skiing was about to transform when his aluminium skis burst on to the competitive scene in 1961. Six years later, the American sports gear manufacturer, Wilson, introduced a steel tennis racket. Head was just as bad at tennis as he was at skiing, so he took over a company called Prince and designed a large composite racket. And then, in 1979, a man named Gary Adams introduced the oxymoronic metal woods to golf and we now have hybrids, or a combination wood–iron, even if they are made of titanium.

It's been a gentle technological revolution, despite wood still being the mandated weapon in cricket and aluminium outlawed in baseball. What Head, who died in 1991, wrought because he was a bum skier set in motion a change in equipment across most sports. Wooden lacrosse sticks have gone the way of leather footballs, which, when wet, could knockout a front row forward if taken flush on the temple.

American historian, Barbara Tuchmann, probably took things a little too far when she wrote, 'In human activity, the invention of the ball may be said to rank with the invention of the wheel.' But it did grease the skids of a social revolution. The reduction in the working week increased leisure time, and the mass marketing of cheaper equipment meant the people picking up clubs and rackets weren't PLUs, or 'People Like Us', as the moneyed classes prefer to call themselves. The dirty fingernail brigade was starting to invade the football fields in America as well. Walter Camp, father of American football and a nineteenth-century coach, once said, 'You don't want your boy "hired" by anyone. If he plays . . . he plays for victory, not for money . . . and he can look you in the eye like a gentleman should.' You get the impression there were no sons of agricultural labourers or factory workers in Camp's teams.

So where did the glorification of the amateur ideal originate? It's generally believed it began with the ancient Olympics, yet they had nothing to do with amateurism. 'Ancient amateurism is a myth', says the classicist David Young in *The Olympic Myth of Greek Amateur Athletics*. This is supported by Andrew Strenk, the official historian of the 1984 Los Angeles Games, who writes, 'The whole concept of amateurism would have been incomprehensible to the ancient Greeks. You had to be a professional to compete in the Olympics, which meant that you had to prove you were a full-time athlete and that you had been doing nothing but training for three months prior to the Games.' Greek athletes were supported by their families during training and first prize was a pair of oxen.

Well, who created the rotten blocks at the foundation of amateurism and had the hide to proclaim it the edifice of sport? Victorian England. The bluebloods who ruled the amateur sports in England's green and pleasant land adopted the concept to keep the lower classes from associating with the upper classes on the fields of play. In the 1870s, the British aristocratic British Amateur Rowing Association separated itself from the oily hands brigade by passing a rule that stated no person is an amateur 'who is or ever has been by trade or employment for wages, a mechanic, artisan or labourer, or engaged in any menial duty'. In other words, the rule barred almost anyone who had ever worked for a living. Since the adoption of that rowing law, writes historian Ronald Smith, in *Sports and Freedom: The Rise of Big-Time College Athletics*, 'Nearly every definition of an amateur in sports has been a negative one . . . Amateurism is not really a moral issue about getting paid or not paid for athletic competition, but is a distinction by class. There is simply no evidence that an amateur is more virtuous than a pro.'

Amateurism created the building blocks through whose crevices crawled the corrupt tennis coaches who demanded appearance money for their starry-eyed Davis Cup players while booking the athletes into sub-standard accommodation and hoarding the secret payments. Brown-paper bag payments were sanctioned at the top, with Australia's Tony Roche once telling me, 'Even in 1966, my best year, when I was allowed to do a private tour of the Caribbean and accept money under the table, I rejoined the Australian team for the French Open and was back on $5 a week.' Ditto the boot money paid rugby union players when the code was amateur. In 1985, when Wallaby great Mark Ella was demoralised with rugby union, he sent a message to St George that he was considering switching codes. We met him in the boardroom of the club and he seemed comfortable with the move, one which would have answered our need for a five eighth. But his agent insisted on trawling the business community for additional sponsorship monies before they could agree to our offer of around $30,000 a year. The top end of town soon heard about the proposed defection, via the private-school educated marketing managers who dominate Sydney companies, and they rallied. 'We sent the hat around and collected enough for a $50,000 a year contract', admits Ross Turnbull, then chairman of the NSWRU.

Amateurism is also responsible for athletes, such as Herb Elliott, being forced to retire at age 21 in order to earn a living. And for those who were denied trophies because someone remembered them being paid one shilling for winning a race at a picnic day for the children of mill workers. Australia's Dawn Fraser, winner of gold medals in the same event at three successive Olympics, was disqualified from her first amateur race at fourteen on the dubious grounds she had been involved with a professional club. She had to stand down from swimming for eighteen months. Another swimmer, Frank Beaurepaire, after competing in the 1908 Olympics, was banned from the 1912 Games because he'd worked as a physical education teacher. He was allowed back for the 1920 show.

The most tragic example of this discrimination against the lesser classes was American Jim Thorpe, who won two gold medals at Stockholm in 1912 but was stripped of them when it was discovered he had received money for competing in a minor baseball game. It took nearly three-quarters of a century for the IOC to right the wrong against a man who was one of the outstanding athletes of the first half century. The medals were returned retrospectively in 1984.

Fortunately, the tradition of paying athletes and swimmers in trinkets and trophies, as if their glory were diminished by something as base as money, has disappeared. It survives as the shamateurism of big-time US college football and basketball, where boosters buy cars for those players successfully recruited and fund sex romps for those being induced to sign declarations of intent. College football and basketball generates billions of dollars in revenue via packed stadiums and TV rights to big bowl games, yet the elite athletes are paid nothing, other than their residential and tuition fees, forcing them to fund their Big-Man-On-Campus lifestyles with gifts from player agents, boosters and gamblers. The agents—many with the most twisted of ethical backbones—get the players' signatures on management contracts that entitle the agents to trailing commissions during long-term and lucrative professional careers.

When the Cold War was fought between Communism and Capitalism, the so-called Free World was in the invidious position of having to compete against athletes masquerading as members of the armed services, but training full-time in sports factories. Even when the United States pulled out of the 1980 Moscow Olympics in protest at the Soviet Union's invasion of Afghanistan (where the now-hated Taliban were backed by the CIA), the USSR was determined to use sport as a vehicle to demonstrate the superiority of their system over the West. The Games were to be a grand coming out party for a nation under siege from rebel neighbours, Afghanistan and Poland. The Soviet Government had spent millions of dollars training athletes and coaches and their officials wanted to ensure their efforts were rewarded.

The field events in the track-and-field program offered the easiest opportunities for blatant corruption. Aware that the tunnelled wind at Lenin Stadium allowed javelin throwers and pole vaulters to throw longer and leap higher, Soviet officials opened the gates when it was time for their athletes to compete. Their athletes won gold and silver in the javelin but a Pole broke the world record in the pole vault, antagonising the jeering crowd by singing Poland's old national anthem at the victory ceremony. The triple jump was rigged to appease an unhappy sponsor but the fix ended in farce when a young Australian made the leap of his life.

This story was initially told to me by David Prince, a silver medallist in the 110-metre hurdles at the 1962 Commonwealth Games and later marketing director of Adidas and president of Athletics Australia. It was subsequently backed up by three of the Moscow competitors themselves.

The 'great shoe-in' began at the Opening Ceremony in Moscow when the USSR's two most-celebrated athletes, Viktor Saneyev, winner of the triple jump at the previous three Olympics, handed the torch to Sergei Belov, captain of the Soviet basketball team, to light the flame. Watching the ritual from the VIP area were IOC president Baron Killanin and Horst Dassler, founder of Adidas and the Baron's close friend, together with the head of Japanese sporting gear company Mizuno. The crowd of 100,000 was spellbound by the mass choirs, ethnic dancers, goosestepping soldiers clutching doves and even a Greek chariot. But the Mizuno chief noted something horribly wrong. Saneyev and Belov were wearing Adidas shoes instead of Mizuno. Mizuno had sponsored the torch relay for US$100,000—outfitting the 3000 torch relay runners as part of a strategy by the traditionally golf- and ski-oriented company to secure a footprint in the lucrative footwear market of the West. The two Soviet athletes, long-term Adidas wearers, were unaware of the embarrassment. The Mizuno boss protested to Killanin who asked Dassler to fix the problem.

The solution was to find an event the Soviets were expected to win, so that the eventual gold medallist would wear Mizuno shoes. An advertising poster would help promote their shoes during the next four years. With Adidas expected to win the men's sprints and long-distance events, and Nike taking the 800 metres and 1500 metres, Dassler decided on the triple jump, where the great Saneyev might win a fourth gold. But the Soviet triple jumpers, having been ordered to wear 'Japanese shoes', turned up for their event wearing Asics, assuming these were the required brand. And a young Australian jumper, Ian Campbell, the top qualifier from the elimination rounds, performed so sensationally in the twelve-man final that he had to be brazenly fouled.

Campbell told me, 'The BBC measured my jump at 17.57 metres, which would have won the event, splitting the Olympic [17.39 metres] and world record [17.89]'. Campbell was fouled for dragging—an arcane rule that prohibits the athlete from scraping the synthetic surface of the runway with his carry leg while executing the middle, or step, phase of the triple jump (an event also known as the 'hop, step and jump'). 'They changed the rules on dragging some years later', said Campbell. 'It was irrelevant anyway, because dragging hinders movement.' Campbell, dispirited, was probably legitimately fouled on his next three jumps, leaving him fifth.

According to a British competitor, Keith Connor, the most blatant injustice was inflicted on a Brazilian, João Carlos de Oliveira, then the world-record holder. He ended up with the bronze medal. 'The most violently robbed guy was the Brazilian', said Connor who finished fourth. 'He was hammering down the runway and jumping 17.50 metres and every time he did it, the red flag went up.' Tragically, de Oliveira had a leg amputated in 1981, the victim of a traffic accident in São Paulo, when a drunken driver ran a red light on a one-way street and smashed into his car. de Oliveira later turned to alcohol and died in 1999 from liver disease.

The gold medal was won by the USSR's Jaak Uudmäe (17.35 metres) ahead of Saneyev (17.24). Saneyev migrated to Sydney in 1991 following the breakup of the Soviet Union and was employed as an assistant jumps coach under Connor, who had also moved to

Australia to become a head coach at the NSW Academy of Sport. Saneyev, too, says he was robbed in 1980. He claims de Oliveira gesticulated excitedly to him after his final jump, waving four fingers. The gesture referred to a fourth gold medal, says Saneyev. 'I knew he did not mean I was fourth placed.' He claims Soviet officials deliberately measured his jump short, a strange decision when he would merely have leap-frogged another Soviet athlete and brought great honour with a fourth gold medal.

Saneyev argues the inflexible Soviet officials had already decided Uudmäe would win because his pre-Olympic form had been better and it would be less risky than setting up a win for Saneyev, who carried an injury into the Games. Connor certainly believes the Soviet Union's bureaucratically strangled hierarchical system didn't allow for any last-minute scope for a final victory-clinching leap by Saneyev. 'By the time of Viktor's last jump, the officials had it all under control and could have given him what they wanted.' Saneyev agrees he wore Adidas shoes to the Opening Ceremony and Asics to the triple jump, saying, 'Mizuno shoes were not good for the triple jump.' Photographs of the event show Uudmäe also in Asics, but a later photograph, professionally shot for a promotional poster, had both Soviet athletes in Mizuno.

By 1988, the 'Free World' had caught up with the Communist bloc at the Olympics—now they had relaxed the rules about paying athletes and had an improved drug regime. However, amateur boxing, the last of the Olympic lilywhites, still persists in refusing to pay its athletes and the results of some of the bouts I have covered at six Games were so violently in contempt of plausibility that I often shuddered involuntarily, as if hit by a straight left. In Seoul in 1988, I witnessed the incredulous, shocked look on the face of American light-middleweight Roy Jones Jnr when his trainer tipped him that the judges had voted 3–2 against him to award the gold medal to his Korean opponent. Jones looked desperately to the skies for justice. When the result was announced, his opponent lifted the American off the floor of the ring as if he were a trophy, conveying the message he joined with almost everyone there in the belief Jones had won. I remember thinking at the time Jones' sense of injustice must have been akin to that of a young Cassius Clay returning from the Rome Olympics with a gold medal. Clay, so the story went, was barred entry to a restaurant in his home town because of the colour of his skin and threw his medal in the nearby river. (Muhammad Ali, as Cassius Clay became known, later admitted inventing the story.)

The year after Seoul, amateur boxing's world body, the International Amateur Boxing Association (AIBA), met in Nairobi and on the agenda was the issue of the three Eastern bloc judges who had taken bribes to defeat Jones. They were suspended for two years, nearly half of which had already passed. By then Jones had turned professional; he went on to be regarded as the best professional boxer—pound for pound, as the old catchphrase goes—in the world.

Evander Holyfield was another subsequent world professional champion who was rorted earlier in his career at the Olympics—at the 1984 Los Angeles Games. He was the best of the 359 boxers in that tournament but, when they gloved up for the finals, Holyfield was back in the bleachers eating a hotdog. In the semifinals, he had met a tattooed New Zealander, Kevin Barry, but was mugged by a Yugoslav referee, Gligorije Novicic. The preceding bout was won by Anton Josipovic, also a Yugoslav. Barry's tactic was to hold Holyfield with one hand while rapping him on the back of the neck with the other. Novicic cautioned Barry and warned him; and then went back to a caution, a no-no in this sport. Near the end of the second round, Holyfield hit Barry with a combination at the precise moment Novicic said, 'Stop.' Barry went down and was out of the Olympics because he had been stopped by a head blow. (It is standard proceedure in Olympic boxing for a boxer stopped by a blow to the head to take no further part in the tournament.) Holyfield went out for hitting on the break. The referee's compatriot, Josipovic, won a gold medal without having anyone to fight.

In the wake of this and widespread scorecard piracy in Los Angeles, together with revelations the judges in Seoul were bribed, amateur boxing introduced an electronic point-scoring system for the Barcelona Olympics. Five judges sit around a ring, each with a computer. If they believe a boxer has landed a clean blow, they press the computer key assigned for that boxer. If three judges press the same key within one second of each other, the system registers a point for the boxer. This system can only be rorted by a judge acting as if he is a monkey at a keyboard, coshing the same key repeatedly and hoping it is matched by two of the other judges. A simple printout of that judge's scoring at the end of the bout would expose him.

So for the next three Games, Olympic boxing had the quality of held-breath but it almost expired following the Athens Games. I spent six months after those 2004 Games researching a scandal which involved accusations that a Sydney referee took instructions from outside the ring, that Mafia figures infiltrated the meetings of referees and judges, and that an Australian heavyweight was robbed of a medal. Australian Olympic Committee president, John Coates, passed on my information to Jacques Rogge when the IOC president visited Brisbane ahead of a meeting in Singapore. According to Coates, Rogge nodded knowingly at the accusations.

He proceeded to charge AIBA with 'betraying athletes.' The IOC imposed a US$12 million freeze on the sport's funding until it improved the judging of bouts, with the strong implication that it should remove the sport's top administration.

The central figure in the Athens scandal was the man who appointed the referees and judges in Athens, Egypt's Dr Ismail Osman. Egyptian boxers won two bronze and one silver medal and, given Egypt had previously won only one boxing medal in Olympic history—a bronze in Rome in 1960—this was the country's best-ever result. Egypt also recorded the highest level of protests in Athens, none of which Dr Osman allowed. Australian heavyweight, Adam Forsyth, lost controversially to an Egyptian, Mohamed Elsayed, in a decision that left fair-minded sportspeople such as former Wallabies captain, John Eales—sitting ringside in his capacity as an AOC athlete liaison officer—dumbfounded. Elsayed, assured of a bronze medal, retired hurt before his next bout.

The worst decision in Athens, though, came when the jury awarded a quarterfinal light heavyweight bout to Egypt's Ahmed Ismail over Greece's Elias Pavlidis. Bottles were thrown into the ring and angry Greek fans stormed the jury, which fled like frightened forest creatures in the face of a bushfire. It was piracy of the worst order—yet another deck chair on the *Titanic* of Olympic boxing. The referee, P.K.M. Raja of India, stopped the bout in the third round with Pavlidis leading 19–12 on the judges' scoring. Pavlidis had a cut above his eye, caused by an elbow from the Egyptian in the second round. Raja should have disqualified Ismail immediately it happened, or at least deducted points. But during the next round, he took Pavlidis to the ring doctor who had no other option but to stop the contest.

When I bombarded Dr Osman in a series of faxes, asking how Ismail could have been declared the winner, he said, 'A protest was presented from Greece concerning an unfair blow from the Egyptian boxer. The committee held a meeting and found the points for Greece were 19–12 but the jury results were 5–0 to Egypt.' (The jury, who sit at a table away from the ringside judges, oversee them, ostensibly as a court of appeal.) In Athens, they served little purpose. Osman also told me, 'It [the jury] also found no intention of the Egyptian boxer to injure the Greek boxer so the committee rejected the protest.' So Pavlidis' four-year hard slog, rising at 4 am to run on an ice-coated road for his home Olympics, were over because the five jurors mysteriously and unanimously had a totally different view of the fight to the judges. Furthermore, the blow, although admitted to be illegal, was ruled unintentional. And Ismail won a bronze medal.

Dr Osman retaliated to my questions about corruption and bribery at Athens by accusing Australian referee/judge Steve Donkin of 'incorrect and shameless behaviour'. Donkin's crime? According to Dr Osman, 'Donkin was getting signals and instructions from some coaches and officials to score points according to whatever comes to him from outside, not according to what was happening in the ring'. Donkin rejected this, saying, 'I've never taken signals off anyone in my life. I'm not sorry for one thing I did at the Olympics. I judged it how I saw it. I was in the top five of officials for six days in a row and then was shafted.'

Donkin was clearly sidelined because he did not produce the required results. A father of three, he was frightened to speak about the Olympics, redirecting questions to his roommate in Athens, Pat Fiacco, then mayor of Regina, Canada. In Athens,

Fiacco had claimed to be so appalled by what he witnessed, he promised Donkin he would take his complaints to the prime minister of Canada. However, when I contacted him, he would not comment on the record.

Referees and judges who attended the sixteen daily meetings in Athens' Peristeri Stadium were gobsmacked at the presence of sinister-looking men in expensive suits with no official role. An atmosphere of fear and intimidation continued months after Athens. 'The Mafia were standing in our meetings every day', one official said. 'They [the IOC] are trying to kick our sport out of the Olympics yet these blokes walk into our meetings and seminars and stand there.' Another long-term official, asked whether some of his younger colleagues were over-dramatising, said, 'Mafia? There were a lot of Russians there, with no official title. One Russian was flashing money every night.' One referee insists he was initially offered US$1000 and then it was increased to US$4000.

After Athens, the AIBA next met in Liverpool, England, and there was a fierce exchange between Dr Osman and the president of Boxing Australia, Sol Spitalnic, over my investigation. The old warhorses eyed each other, with the Egyptian saying provocatively, 'What do you think of my responses to the questions from Australia?' Spitalnic, a Jewish businessman from Melbourne who sat comfortably in an essentially Muslim-run sport, warned Dr Osman, saying, 'Don't take me on.' The meeting sniffed something important and demanded to know the basis of the seething exchange. The 82-year-old AIBA president, Anwar Chowdhry, was forced to intervene. Chowdhry, a retired Pakistani engineer, was wheelchair bound and very alert. Boxing officials spoke admiringly of his drinking capacity. He celebrated his 80th birthday twice—in both Turkey and Egypt—and then chaired an

AIBA meeting from 9 am to 5 pm. Chowdhry adjourned the Liverpool meeting while his son-in-law, the AIBA secretary, raced away and returned with printed copies of my questions and Dr Osman's responses.

Six delegates of EABA, the powerful European division of AIBA, acted immediately on the material, resolving to remove those 'who were orchestrating the unfair results [in Athens]'. The EABA delegates also petitioned AIBA to fall in line with an IOC request to allow officials to work at successive Olympics. Chowdhry, who insisted on being called 'Professor', had introduced a rule barring officials who had officiated at one Olympics from refereeing/judging at the next Games. Ostensibly, it was designed to stop corrupt judges/referees from backing-up, an admission judging was corrupt. But maybe Chowdhry knew what he was doing. An expert on the matter, Arthur Tunstall—when told Chowdhry's reason for the rule—said, 'It is the most ridiculous rule I have heard in 60 years in the sport. You can control them better when they are novices.' Chowdhry, Dr Osman and their lieutenants eventually lost their positions at the next world conference of AIBA: the IOC restored funding and there were no reports of bias at the Beijing Olympics.

The mid twentieth century was the pivot on which sport turned, leaving noble amateurs like Dr Roger Bannister, the first man to break the four-minute mile, and Sir Edmund Hillary, the first to climb Mount Everest, as rearguards for the past. It wasn't just that amateurism was in retreat, everything was changing. Sport would become more about personal milestones than team achievements, more about celebrities than heroes, more about gamesmanship than sportsmanship.

It would seem no sport is immune from accusations of match fixing—even lawn bowls. The New Zealand mens four was accused of deliberately losing a match against Thailand at the August 2009 Asia-Pacific Championship in Malaysia. Canada and World Bowls both claimed the Kiwi team underperformed, forcing Bowls New Zealand to hold an inquiry—New Zealand's loss meant Canada didn't make the playoffs. The Kiwi bowlers countered by saying the whole sport of lawn bowls was corrupt and New Zealand management was solely concerned with making money. 'We didn't throw the game', one of the Kiwi bowlers said, 'we just lost. It happens occasionally.' He then proceeded to blame his coach for creating the drama, saying, 'He should be charged with impersonating a coach.'

While, personal jealousies and egos will always promote false accusations, there can be little doubt over another case of cheating that surfaced at the same time as 'Bowlsgate'. The *London Times* called it 'the worst single piece of cheating in world sport'. It distinguished itself from simple cheating, as in a schoolboy taking crib notes into the exam. This was a case of the teacher supplying the model answers to the pupil.

Formula 1 driver, Nelson Piquet Jr, the son of the eponymous three-times world champion, blew the whistle on a crash that had been deliberately staged at the 2008 September Grand Prix in Singapore. Piquet, sacked by his Renault team for failing to produce the results they needed, retaliated by exposing the 'accident' he was told to have, which had allowed his teammate, Fernando Alonso, to win. Alonso, who began the Singapore race in fifteenth position, had an unusual early pit stop, allowing him to fill up; and then Piquet 'crashed' into a wall. Crashes have potentially lethal consequences in an already dangerous sport, yet

Renault staged one. Out came the safety car, which meant all cars were required to follow it, without overtaking each other. One by one, however, the other drivers pulled out to fill their tanks, allowing Alonso to slowly move up the grid to first place and win his first race in a year.

After Piquet made public his revelations, Renault sacked the team's managing director, the playboy Italian Flavio Briatore. The International Automobile Federation (FIA) handed Renault a suspended ban for a year, effectively meaning the sanction would only be imposed if they did it again. FIA obviously blamed Briatore, who was given an 'unlimited' ban, presumably preventing him participating in the sport for life. Bernie Ecclestone, despite holding the commercial rights to Formula 1, could not help his great friend and co-owner of soccer club, Queens Park Rangers. It was a show of strength from Max Mosley, then in his sixteenth and final year as FIA head. The previous year Mosley had admitted to participating in sadomasochistic sex with five prostitutes but won a defamation action against a London tabloid that said those participating in the sessions wore Nazi memorabilia. Mosley's father was leader of the British fascists during World War II.

If this episode of filling up with petrol early in the race gave a new meaning to 'tanking', it's been practised in its conventional form in the AFL for years. Conspiring to lose is a difficult task in a team sport but the AFL manages it. For years, the AFL has denied teams deliberately lose end-of-regular season matches in order to win high draft choices from the rookie list, under a scheme where the best young player in the nation goes to the worst team in the nation. When Richmond coach Terry Wallace admitted, after being sacked in 2009, to doing nothing to alter the course of a Round 22 match in 2005 against St Kilda, the AFL dismissed his comments. Richmond lost to St Kilda by ten points and earned a priority pick in the draft.

A Melbourne Demons player, Russell Robertson, who finished with the club at the end of the 2009 season, attended a grand final lunch in Tasmania where he made some startling admissions. His club ran last and received the prized priority picks, who would not be available in subsequent seasons because the best talent was quarantined for the planned new clubs, Gold Coast and Western Sydney. Robertson was quoted as saying, 'I'm not saying we tanked, I'm just saying players were played out of position. We've got a centre-half forward playing in the ruck, we've got our backline playing in the forward line, we've got our forward line playing in the backline. It's not hard to figure it out. You can't blame the coach. It is more just the way the AFL is at the moment . . .'

When the Victorian Commission for Gambling Regulation wrote to the AFL asking for evidence that teams did not tank late-season matches, the AFL did not initially reply, requiring a second letter to be sent. Supporters of cellar-dweller clubs in the AFL have actually become inured to their team losing in August, eyeing off the prized recruits who they hope will rebuild their team.

Badminton's showpiece event—the All England Championships—was marred in 2009 by match fixing by the Chinese team. The defending men's champion retired from the semi final, giving the Olympic champion an easy path to the final where the well-rested Chinese competitor destroyed his Malaysian opponent. China has long been accused of taking advantage of its large numbers of competitors to rig matches and manipulate world rankings so the maximum number of Chinese competitors qualify for a tournament.

Horse racing has been plagued with race-fixing scandals, including the ludicrous swap of the better performing horse Bold Personality for the lesser Fine Cotton in a 1500-metre race in Brisbane in August 1984. It was an amateurish sting, including a splash of white paint on the horse's legs in the backyard of a house near the Eagle Farm course. When the trainer realised he had been too lavish with the Dulux, he bandaged the horse's forelegs. Meanwhile, in Sydney, race touts, aware of the sting, gossiped in the betting ring. They included an Irish priest, Father O'Dwyer, who was already infamous for raffling a grand piano in a parish fundraiser without the permission of the owner (who, when he learned of the prize, was told, 'Don't worry, you'll win the raffle'). Not surprisingly, the stewards were on to it before Fine Cotton passed the winning post.

But how many horses fail to run on their merits and who is to know? When a trainer tells a jockey 'give him a run', he is not telling the hoop to let the horse have his head. It's almost an Orwellian reversal of meaning, in that this is actually a euphemism for ordering the jockey to pull the horse up. Gear changes offer a grab bag of opportunities, with tongue ties, blinkers and glued shoes all influencing a horse's performance.

Match fixing is corrupt, as opposed to gamesmanship which the bow-tied essayists will argue took over from sportsmanship when athletes began being paid. No sport is exempt from gamesmanship of some kind. Kenya's marathon runners were so well-known for knocking the paper cups full of water off the drinks tables set at regular intervals over the course that Australia's Robert de Castella had to come up with a counter strategy at the 1982 Commonwealth Games in Brisbane. A track-and-field official told me 'Deek' positioned an army of helpers at the tables along the course, with each one handing him an opened bottle as he approached. I later put this to Deek, who agreed the Kenyans were not above tipping over the drinks but added, 'If you took an open bottle from anyone, you'd be mad'.

Even sealed bottles can cause problems. 'I'm still convinced my drink was spiked in the 1987 marathon in Rome', he said. 'My legs just stopped after I took a drink at the twenty-kilometre mark. I couldn't lift my legs. The family we were staying with in Italy said it was the work of Mafia.' At the same world championships, the result of the winning long jump was posted the instant the Italian leapt into the pit.

President Clinton was accused of not only cheating on his wife but in golf as well. Some men would consider Clinton's habit of taking 'mulligans' (a free second attempt when the first shot is unsatisfactory) more heinous than his two-timing Hillary. John Dryden, the English poet, wrote: 'When I consider life, 'tis all a cheat / yet, fooled with hope, men favour the deceit.' In 1999, two birds were expelled from Sweden's national pigeon-racing championships after they tested positive to cortisone, a banned substance. Even TV networks cheat. When twitchers complained to US giant CBS that they'd heard geographically inappropriate species chirping in the background of some of the sports telecasts, the network admitted that it sometimes played taped birdsongs for 'ambient sound'.

Where does cheating end and gamesmanship begin? The NFL team, the New England Patriots, during a 1982 game, had one swath of their field snowploughed (by a parolee), helping them to kick a fourth-quarter field goal in a 3–0 win over the Miami Dolphins. It was the first time that a levelling of the playing field had exactly the opposite effect. Sometimes, athletes don't have to say much to affect a result. During the Australian swimming championships in Adelaide in the lead-up to the 1990 Commonwealth Games in Auckland, Lisa Curry-Kenny made a comeback. The muscled mother intimidated the fifteen-year-old girls in the change room simply by undressing in front of them.

The week before the 2003 world surfing title was to be decided at Pipeline in Hawaii, the greatest rivalry of the modern era erupted. The detached, disciplined Kelly Slater had gone into self-imposed exile from the pro tour after his sixth world title in 1998. When he eventually returned, he found his good friends had retired and in their place was the volatile Kauaian, Andy Irons. Competitors at Pipeline rented team houses lining the beach on Oahu's North Shore and Slater simply walked into Iron's house unannounced, claiming to be looking for another surfer for a game of golf. 'Kelly walked in, took a look around and just split,' an observer said. 'Andy was a bit shook up by the unexpected visitor, saying, "What the fuck was that?"' A few days later a slanging match developed between them on the water, with Irons saying, 'Game fucking on.' When they both made the Pipeline final, the year's points tally meant the winner would take the world title. Before they paddled out, Slater sauntered across to Irons, draped his arm across his shoulders, and said, 'I love you, man.' The tactic failed—Irons won the world championship.

Coaches make a Jesuitical distinction between violent play and 'controlled aggression,' meaning what is illegal to one person is tactics to another. When I coached the first-grade Western Suburbs rugby league team, we were accused of being violent, rather than overly physical. Yet our explosive beginnings to matches was a con in itself. Opposition teams spent 80 minutes trying to square up for the earlier violence, while we quickly reverted to playing good football.

The brutality of water polo is played out largely beneath the surface of the water, where the testicle grabbing, back clawing and general mayhem that takes place makes a rugby union scrum look genteel. Nor is it exactly a tea party above the waterline, with players bobbing in the water like corks and matches ending in confusion and controversy. The whole game seems predicated on trying to impress the referee you are not committing an illegality when you are, and convincing the referee the opposition is fouling, when they are not.

Much of the brutality has been legislated out of the football codes owing to the many-headed hydra of TV cameras, to the extent that players are more likely to take a dive than throw a straight left. A striker in soccer seems to play two positions—centre forward and prone. Defenders prance around, make contact and then collapse in agony, re-enacting the death scene from *Othello* in order to attract a penalty. Sport's greatest prize, the FIFA World Cup, was won in 2006 by an Italian player taking a dive after receiving a head-butt to the chest from the French captain. Italy's Marco Materazzi persisted in tugging Zinedine Zidane's shirt, prompting the Frenchman to say, 'If you want my shirt so much, I'll give it to you afterwards.' Materazzi responded with a remark to the effect he would prefer Zidane's sister, or mother. It prompted a head butt so gentle it would be called a love tap in rugby league and the French captain was red-carded.

The faking of injuries at soccer's 2010 World Cup in South Africa was so pathetic, Australian commentators referred to the number of players collapsing on the turf as the 'death toll.' Yellow cards handed to the perpetrators of these foul deeds were dubbed 'resurrections', based on the speed with which the wounded player regained his feet.

Brazil's performance in the final of the 1998 FIFA World Cup has never been satisfactorily explained. Their best player, Ronaldo, was not named on the original team sheet and rumours circulated he had suffered food poisoning. He was a very late inclusion in the team and performed well below his best in the 3–0 loss to host nation France. He later said, somewhat mysteriously, 'We lost the World Cup, but I won another cup . . . my life'.

France was also the beneficiary of an illegality missed by match officials when French captain Thierry Henry's 'hand of frog' caused his counry to progress to the 2010 World Cup in South Africa, while Ireland missed out. Henry handled the ball in the lead-up to team mate William Gallas' equaliser that gave France a 1–1 draw and a 2–1 aggregate win. The French striker later admitted he regretted his post-goal celebration but revealed he felt let down by his own national federation who did not contact him for a couple of days. Henry also demonstrated some neat footwork when he said a replay against Ireland would be the fairer solution—but he offered this only after FIFA declared the result would stand. Soccer has resisted calls for a video review of goals, possibly because it knows it would open a Pandora's Box of egregious diving if replays were extended to general play.

Rugby league coaches know that if play has stopped and a player is prone, the video referee will take the opportunity to review the action and possibly find some accidental contact he deems to be illegal. Players are therefore instructed to stay down, hoping to milk a penalty. This is alien to many players, particularly those brought up under the credo 'never show 'em you're hurt'. I recall the 2006 NRL grand final eliminator between the Bulldogs and the Broncos. The match swung on a penalty the Broncos were awarded, despite the Bulldogs' Sonny Bill Williams being felled by a wicked blow. Had Williams stayed down, the video referee would have detected the illegality and the Bulldogs would have been awarded a penalty; thus Brisbane may not have proceeded to the grand final which they won. Three months after the grand final, I met Sonny Bill and congratulated him, while asking why he did not stay down. 'My father would have killed me if I did', he said.

A rugby union winger playing for the Harlequins club in England was suspended for twelve months after he faked an injury by biting on a capsule so he could leave the field with a bleeding mouth. His exit allowed a kicker to come on and attempt a field goal. Signficantly, the capsule was purchased at a joke shop near Clapham Junction. But the sport's bosses weren't impressed, banning Harlequins director of rugby for three years. But this sport appears reluctant to outlaw deliberate stoppages; it appears to be compulsory in rugby union for a big fat bloke to sit down where a scrum is being packed so as to slow the game down. The AFL has moved in the opposite direction and implemented measures to speed things up—yet the desperate scramble of players for the ball, involving players piling on top of each other, sometimes makes the code resemble rugby union.

Rugby league has oscillated between periods when the game is too quick and too slow. Gang tackling slowed things down, with the defence holding the ball carrier upright and waiting to be joined by two or more fellow tacklers in a bizarre tactic called "dancing". They would then collapse in a bad soufflé of bodies, each peeling off slowly while their defensive line was reset. Eventually this was countered by the surrender tackle, where the ball carrier would dive at the feet of the defence in order to avoid the monstering and so he could rise quickly to his feet and play the ball. But this, in turn, led to repetitive running from dummy half, advantaging the attack. The counter was the grapple tackle, a martial arts-type grip on the throat, cutting off the wind supply—a ball carrier gasping for breath is more likely to be concerned for his life than worried about a fast play-the-ball. By 2009, the NRL had countered this with two referees—one standing over the ruck to detect grapple tackles and 'chicken wings' (where arms are prised back forcing the ball carrier to release the ball) and the other monitoring the defensive line.

The battle between the rule breakers and rule makers is proceeding in AFL as well, where the code is doing everything it can to combat its most feared enemy: soccer. The 'bump'—a unique aspect of the game, where a defender collides with a player supporting the ball carrier—is now punishable if any contact is made with the head, albeit accidental, because the code will do anything to demonstrate to mothers that kids can't get hurt playing AFL. The AFL is desperate to restore their famous 'speccy', where a player leaps high above the pack for the ball, but coaches, more concerned about retaining possession, instruct their players to kick backwards and waste time. In this sense, the AFL has achieved its aim because their game sometimes resembles soccer.

Each ANZAC Day, in the hours before the contest, coaches relate graphic stories of the bravery of Gallipoli and, in a fine disregard for history and geography, they quote World War II US General George 'Blood and Guts' Patton; and yet we're entitled to wonder whether the gamesmanship on display is more the reverse of the ANZAC legend. Across the codes, players collapse when not hit; they persistently kick short to an unmarked player to avoid contested situations; they kick backwards to waste time; in league, the water carriers even stand with the defence, creating the impression there is an extra defender in the line. When teams are accused of such tactics, they protest this is merely propaganda by a beaten opposition. In other words, on our football pitches we are witnesses to military tactics designed to avoid meeting the enemy man-on-man, or to deceive him, or accusations of breaches of a type of Geneva Convention. In fact, we're entitled to ask whether the collective football codes and war have changed places in a ludicrous parody of each other.

When the United States blundered into Iraq, this was similar to the bull-like charges of an old front rower; but on the other hand, the four codes in Australia in the late "noughties" appeared as if they had become games of falling down, kicking backwards, surrendering at the feet of the opposition and generally avoiding contact. 'Some teams look like the Italian army in World War II', one NRL coach admitted, an allusion to ethnic stereotyping by TV personality David Frost, who once joked that 1939–45 Italian tanks had four reverse gears and one forward gear, 'The forward gear, in case the enemy attacked from the rear', Frost explained.

Technology has compromised sport at all levels, from the spying scandals in Formula 1 racing to the polyurethane swimsuits worn at the world championships in Rome in 2009. Formula 1 team McLaren was fined $120 million and waved out of the constructor's championship after being caught with a 780-page Ferrari dossier. McLaren had been receiving a systematic flow of information from a spy within rival Ferrari for nearly three months in 2008. The information on brakes, weight distribution, aerodynamic balance and tyre inflation came to McLaren's chief designer from Ferrari's chief mechanic.

The 'non-textile' swimsuits, introduced in 2008, led to a glut of world records in Rome, with many swimmers shaving seconds off their personal bests. In yet another muddled-headed response by a sport's administrator, world swimming's governing body, FINA, announced that the swimsuits would be banned in 2010. The world's swimming champions in Rome were allowed to keep their titles, while FINA retained the sponsorships from the swimsuit manufacturers. Yet by the end of October 2009, 200 world records had fallen since the suits were introduced. The only record to withstand the invasion of the bodysuits was the 1500-metre time set at the World Championships in Fukuoka, Japan, in 2001 by Australia's Grant Hackett. Murray Rose, who broke fifteen world records in his career, equated the flood of best times with the drug-fuelled rush of Eastern European track-and-field records in the 1980s. 'Except the gap is even wider', said Rose. He declared swimming had been 'trashed' by the high-tech suits. 'I don't know whether FINA always has the swimmers' interests at heart', he lamented.

It's not as if FINA officials weren't warned of the impact of the suits. In January, 2009, Grant Stoelwinder, the coach of Australian sprinter Eamon Sullivan, was quoted as saying, 'The suits do make a difference and now we are getting to the point where some suits are starting to make a lot more of a difference'. Five months later, German Olympic champion Britta Steffen said of the new swimsuit she wore to break the world 100-metre freestyle record of Australia's Libby Trickett, 'I felt like a speed boat in water and never in my life would I have believed that a human being could glide like that'. Yet in the face of all this evidence,

FINA simply trod water, seemingly powerless to act. I suspect swimming's old guard—former champions like Rose—probably forced some action, angry their old marks were being erased with such ease.

Some sports, such as American football, succumb to the arms race, allowing all types of technology to invade the playing field. Wide receivers were the first to wear special gloves, resulting in the taking of some spectacular catches. Today, players in other positions, such as running backs, also wear gloves. By contrast, one of the few American innovations allowed in the rugby codes in Australia is the use of kicking tees. My view is all innovations should be allowed provided they don't injure opponents. The ice hockey type shoulder pads worn by Bulldogs players in the mid 1980s certainly stung tacklers.

Sledging has become common in all sports. Because the term came into currency in Australia in the 1970s, it is often assumed that abusive language in sport began with the Chappell era. Ian Chappell, the Australian cricket captain from 1971–75, resents this reputation, claiming that it has been written by so many journalists it has become a self-perpetuating myth. Chappell's teams, particularly those that included fast bowler Dennis Lillee, have acquired a reputation akin to a motorbike gang in creams. 'Chappelli' told me, 'It really pisses me off that Australia in general and my era in particular have been loaded with this misinterpretation. Abuse of cricketers has been about for a long time. For England to suggest we started it is wrong. Their accusation ignores Freddie Trueman [English fast bowler of the 1950s] who used some very colourful language. Most English county batsmen would have copped some abuse from Fiery Fred over time.'

Chappell can put a definite date on the occasion the term 'sledge' entered the cricket lexicon: 'It was during the 1964–65 Sheffield Shield season in Adelaide and had absolutely nothing to do with what happened on the field. New South Wales was playing my team, South Australia, and, as was the usual practice, both teams had this huge party in the motel room of Graeme Corling [NSW right-arm swing bowler]. Corling was a bloke who dropped the magic word in front of everybody, well before it became fashionable to do so. His nickname was "I'llbe" from the song, "I'll Be Calling You". Eventually the party broke up and there were only four of us left in I'llbe's room. A New South Wales player came back to the room with a sheila. He asked, "What happened to the party?" I'llbe said, "The party's all fucked up". The New South Wales player was embarrassed and said, "I'llbe, you're as subtle as a sledgehammer". From that incident, anyone who swore in front of a woman became known as a "sledge". About this time, the Percy Sledge number, "When A Man Loves A Woman", became popular. A man who swore in front of a woman became a "Percy" or a "sledge". The next generation of players, or the media, thought it referred to language on the field.' And so a batsman would return to the dressing room after getting out and warn his team mates, saying, 'There is a bit of Percy Sledge going on out there today.'

Initially, sledging was mainly confined to fast bowlers. If fieldsmen began idle chatter, batsmen would refuse to face up until they shut up. Though Chappell deplored mindless talk, he justified aggressive behaviour by fast bowlers, saying, 'A weakness of character is as legitimate a target as a weakness outside the off stump.' Because tests are played over five days, cricket is a game where a player with a hidden psychological problem is soon smoked out.

The most effective counter to sledging is to force the fielding team to laugh. Zimbabwean tail-end batsman Eddo Brandes once frustrated Australian pace bowler Glenn McGrath, who could not get him out. McGrath walked up to Brandes and asked, 'How come you're so fat?' Brandes instantly replied, 'Because every time I fuck your wife, she gives me a biscuit'. Similarly, England's Jimmy Ormond was met at the crease with the comment from Australia's Mark Waugh, twin brother of captain Steve, 'What are you doing here? There's no way you're good enough to play for England?' Ormond replied, 'Maybe not but at least I'm the best player in my family'.

The ICC responded to the public outcry over sledging during the volatile Australia–India test series of 2007–8, announcing 'a zero tolerance' approach, devolving the responsibility to umpires. 'The umpire seeking to lay a charge shall be required to take into account the context of the particular situation and whether the words or gesture are likely to be regarded as obscene, or give offence, or insult another person', the ICC missive read. It was a bureacrat's response to a cultural problem. It added to the already onerous responsibilities on umpires, all of whom are neutral in Test matches and therefore without intimate knowledge of the cultural sensitivities of either team. How are they to judge what is obscene, offensive or merely humorous repartee? Players responded to the announcement by declaring it could render the game boring and lead to dobbing!

The equivalent term for sledging in the United States is 'trash talk', and it means the same: insulting language used to upset or intimidate; hot words to make the opponent lose his cool. It's common in basketball but is declining in the football codes, not because of political correctness or players' newfound respect for each other, but because of the increasing speed of the game. The reduction in stoppages in some sports and the overall increase in the fitness of players and referees has muzzled the sledgers. They simply don't have the oxygen to maintain a barrage of abuse.

Furthermore, the language of players is often interpreted as sledging when in fact it is often shorthand communication to alert a team mate to a desperate situation. When a footballer yells out, 'Watch the black bloke', it can be a cry to a fellow defender warning him of a clever Aboriginal fullback lurking on the blindside ready to take a pass. Similarly, 'Get the fat cunt' can refer to an overweight front-row forward, or 'Blood nut will get it' means a red-headed player is poised to receive the ball. These are comments directed to the most obvious physical characteristic of the opponent, rather than an attack on his race, weight or complexion. Again, humour is the antidote. The great aboriginal AFL player 'Polly' Farmer remembers someone once yelling out, 'You're nothing but a bloody nigger'. Polly said, 'I yelled back, "No, I'm not. I'm a brilliant nigger".' In more leisurely sports, such as golf, sledging is subtle with a veneer of humour, such as the endless chatter of Lee Trevino. Close encounters of the word kind are common in all sports and all countries. They certainly pre-date the Chappell era.

So how much has tennis changed since Jack Kramer's day? The term 'sisterectomy' was coined to describe the phenomenon, notable during the early careers of the Williams sisters, by which one of them, Venus or Serena, would remove herself from a match for the benefit of the other. But what tennis player hasn't surrendered a set when his serve has been broken early in order to fortify himself physically and mentally for the next? Tennis

Australia has heavy punishments for match fixing, including fifteen year jail terms, and yet ATP officials are culpable. They changed the ranking system from one where a player automatically slipped down the rankings if he lost a tournament in round one to a 'best of' arrangement where a player's results from, say, fourteen tournaments are averaged.

If a player were to conspire with his Round 1 opponent to lose a tournament, he stands to gain four ways. Firstly, he collects the Round 1 losing payment. Secondly, his agreement with his opponent could involve receiving the winner's payment as well—after all, the first-round winner will pick up a bigger cheque in Round 2, even if he loses. Thirdly, via a friend, the first-round loser can place a huge bet on himself to lose with Betfair, whose online betting exchange seeks to match two punters—one who wagers the player will win and another who says he will lose. Alternatively, he can back his opponent with any number of corporate bookmakers around the world. Fourthly, he can ask for a release from the tournament following his Round 1 demise and head off immediately to another potentially more lucrative event somewhere else in the world—if he wins in Round 1 at the next tournament, his ranking points could rise. Even if he doesn't conspire with his Round 1 opponent, he merely misses out on that cheque and no-one ever knows the final double fault in the 6–4, 6–4 loss was deliberate.

Choking, or the failure to perform under pressure, afflicts all athletes, but tennis players are particularly vulnerable. Unless it's doubles, there are no team mates to help absorb the stress or the blame. There's no clock to run out. No coasting, or sitting on the ropes, or kicking for touch. Play conservatively and your opponent will sense it and drive the ball down your throat. Tennis' most memorable choker was Jana Novotna, who double-faulted when she was within a point of taking a 5–1 lead over Steffi Graf in the final at Wimbledon in 1993. Graf won the match and Novotna wept during the presentation, resting her head on the shoulder of the Duchess of Kent. She was cruelly called 'No-no Novotna, the lady from Chokeoslovakia'. However, it's not as if Wimbledon was her only meltdown. She squandered an even more commanding lead in the third round of the French Open in 1995. Her coach, Hana Mandliková, when asked to explain Novotna's mental disintegation, said, 'You can be too intelligent', meaning she over-complicated things with too much thought, rather than allowing instinct and reaction to take over.

Yet if a high IQ was the culprit here, I wondered during a long interview with golfer Greg Norman whether maybe the reverse was his problem. We met at Port Douglas in February 1990, after he had been criticised for his conservative play on the final hole of the 1989 US Masters. Instead of winning a green jacket, he looked like he was playing in a straightjacket—he needed only a par to gain a playoff with the eventual winner, Nick Faldo, but his five-iron approach plunged metres short of the green. At the 72nd hole of the 1986 Masters, his six iron had gone right and he'd also bogeyed. Add Fuzzy Zoeller's beating him in an 18-hole playoff at the 1984 US Open and Bob Tway's bunker shot for a birdie on the last hole of the 1986 PGA and I had to ask Norman if he was a choker. He dismissed it in a Greek tragedian way, saying, 'The other guys want to beat you so bad that things happen'.

Okay, bad luck has contributed to Norman's record of having won only two majors. Who would have expected Larry Mize to chip in from 42 metres to defeat him on the second hole of a sudden-death playoff at the 1987 Masters? Also, at the 1990 British Open, in the first-ever four-hole playoff in the history of the majors, the rules stated the golfers would play holes one and two and end with the 17th and 18th. Norman birdied the first hole while his opponents made pars. If this had been the Masters or the PGA, with their sudden-death playoffs, Norman would have been preparing his acceptance speech. But on the final hole he hit a drive that found previously undiscovered hazards and Mark Calcavecchia joined the growing list of golfers who have been bravely congratulated by Norman on the final hole of a major.

In 1990, I found Norman too ingenuous to be mentally tough. He turned 35 while in Port Douglas and had a spectacular food-fight with fellow golfer Curtis Strange during his birthday party. This was a time when Africa was suffering mass starvation and Freedom From Hunger advertisements were everywhere. Earlier, at Port Lincoln, 'The Great White Shark' attracted criticism from the environmentalists because his fishing expedition went dangerously close to a seal colony. He boasted at a press conference about the TV footage of him in a steel cage enraging white pointers by teasing them with tuna bait.

He also upset many people, particularly women, when he declared he would have won twice as many majors had he met and married former tennis player Chris Evert earlier. This should be considered in the context of what he told me in Port Douglas about his then wife, Laura: 'She's my eyes and my ears outside my body. Laura's not only my wife, she's my best friend. She's the one I listen to. I take advice from her and it helps a lot.' Norman's marriage to Evert was over in nine months.

In 2009, I was at odds with my colleagues at the *Sydney Morning Herald* over a story which appeared after NRL team the Roosters lost to the Cowboys in the final round match. The Roosters led 16–6 at half-time but lost 32–16. There had been newspaper speculation before the game that the Roosters would lose by thirteen points or more. The bookies squealled before and after the match, although the size of the payout was not significant. I watched the match live. I concluded, at the time, the Roosters gave up when the Cowboys were twelve points ahead and seven minutes were left on the clock. But I don't believe they conspired to lose. Why take a sixteen point lead and make it hard for yourself if you intend to lose? Furthermore, it was the final game of their great stalwart, Craig Fitzgibbon. It would have been gross disrespect to cheat in the game that sent him to retirement. In any case, the unfit Roosters had been fading at the end of games for two months.

The newpaper speculation the players had read earlier in the day became a self-fulfilling prophesy. The body language of footballers is hard to read. Other than the players themselves, the best people to interpret it accurately are coaches. Journalists tapping at keyboards in the press room usually can't tell the difference between uncommitted and exhausted play. Sometimes a game spirals out of control, gathering a momentum all of its own and everyone is powerless to stop it. It's like stepping into a grave.

Of course, what some see as cheating is, in fact, choking. 'The thing about tennis,' says John McEnroe, 'Is that no matter what happens, you have to win the last point. It's called choking for a reason.' As the former 'Superbrat' says, 'Sometimes you really feel like you can hardly breath.'

McEnroe's countryman, Andre Agassi, made a comment in his book, *Open*, which echoed the words expressed earlier in this chapter by Pancho Gonzales. Agassi suggested tanking was 'almost harder than winning.' He was referring to a semi-final match against fellow American Michael Chang at the Australian Open in 1996. Agassi admitted throwing the match to avoid meeting the man he loathed, Boris Becker, in the final. Nicknamed 'The Showman', Agassi appeared on the point of tears at the Melbourne press conference after his 6–1, 6–4, 7–6 loss. Yet of tennis writers, he observed in his memoirs: 'They never get it right. When I tank, they say I'm not good enough; when I'm not good enough, they say I tank.'

FIVE
FURTHER

Maybe it was the arrival of Muhammad Ali that shattered forever the brittle belief that sport existed apart from the rest of society. It was Ali, resplendent in his contrived egotism, political conviction and racial pride, who showed how much sport is inextricably intertwined with the great issues of our time—war, race, politics, religion. His daughter, also a boxer, added gender equality to that list.

My personal experience of the US version of the role of Sport As The Glue Of Life was in 1993; it was the replay in New York of the NFL's 'greatest ever game'. The original match had been played on 28 December 1958 at Yankee Stadium between the New York Giants and the Indianapolis Colts. It was the first overtime result in NFL history—the match was tied after regular time and then went to extra time, or what rugby league calls 'golden point', when the Colts won 23–17.

The 35th anniversary match was unremarkable and certainly did not reach the heights of the fabled contest played in 1958. However, the bus trip back from Giants Stadium in the Meadowlands mirrored the best of American life. It was a mobile melting pot of African-Americans (or blacks, which was then the acceptable term, having replaced Negroes), whites, Hispanics, females,

males, young and old. It was also a pleasurable trip down memory lane.

Someone discovered that the kindly man in the fur-lined coat sitting halfway back was Y.A. Tittle, the Giants quarterback when they won three Eastern Division titles in the 1960s. Everyone began excitedly chatting and someone introduced Y.A. to the reporter from Australia. Y.A. then made a comment about the attention he had received, an observation which should resonate with all long-term players and coaches: 'They love you in the beginning, hate you in the middle and love you in the end.' Fans traditionally welcome a new coach/player to their club, confident he can work miracles; then revile him when he doesn't deliver multiple premierships. Then they cry when he leaves. (St George's coterie of passionate female supporters farewelled my coaching career there by presenting me with a red-and-white cock-sock, the amount of wool used neither matching reality, nor their grand expectations for the team.)

Giants fans are passionate supporters and included Jimmy Hoffa, the New York mobster from the 1960s who is rumoured to be buried in one of the end zones of the Meadowlands stadium. 'Jimmy never misses a home game', one of the Giants fans quipped. But the anniversary match was also a snapshot of the past and the future. Y.A. evoked memories of a time when it was good to be square in the sense of square meals, square deals and square jaws. The standard American quarterback back then had flat-topped hair, blue eyes, called older males 'Sir' and was white. At half-time, the old players from the 1958 game were introduced to the crowd and, despite the long coats wrapping these aged warriors, it was clear the colour differential was two to one, white to black. Yet the ratio of the ones actually playing that day was one white to two blacks. In other words, in a generation the racial balance had reversed.

Okay, in 1958 the decision-makers—the head coaches and the quarterbacks—were white while the labourers and those in speedy positions were predominantly black. To some, the NFL in 1958 must have resembled a 1970s map of Africa: white governments and black workers. But thirty years later—at the 26 January 1988 Super Bowl in San Diego—the Washington Redskins, with the NFL's first black quarterback, humiliated the Denver Broncos. I also attended that match, especially significant because I managed, via the time difference, to have two consecutive Australia Days. Today, black head coaches and quarterbacks are no longer rare in the NFL, with the 2009 winning Super Bowl team, the Pittsburgh Steelers, coached by an African-American.

It would be tempting to conclude that sport in the United States is the high road to upward social mobility, an escape from the ghetto, but there are many illogical angles to this oft-expressed view. It implies a large proportion of the black community has deliberately set itself the goal of providing gladiators for white arenas. It also symbolically says blacks are so devoid of dignity, that they can be rescued only by becoming popular sports figures. Or, that a black athlete with 'super-human' skill can win the same normal decencies an ordinary white man takes for granted, provided he takes the sports route.

When an African-American schooled in the public education system is elected President of the United States, perhaps we can say social equality is on the horizon. No wonder, therefore, when Barack Obama was inaugurated as president, Lonni Ali, wife of Muhammad 'The Greatest' Ali, told her husband, 'I do believe you have just been surpassed'. Ali was the sui generis athlete of my generation—the black heavyweight boxer who could outwit white people at upmarket dinner parties, on topics from art to escargots. Even when he failed the intelligence test for induction to the US Army, he had an answer to the rednecks who reviled him as an 'uppity nigger': 'I only said I was the greatest, not the smartest.' But his fans always believed he deliberately failed the test, motivated by his pacifist politics. He was reviled for saying, 'No Viet Cong ever called me a nigger', but today the US trades with a united Vietnam led by the 'Viet Cong' and most Americans now concede the war was wrong.

Ali didn't fit the stereotype advanced by African-American social philosopher, Shelby Steele. Steele divides prominent African-Americans into 'challengers', such as civil rights activist Jesse Jackson and intimidating filmmaker Spike Lee—people who assume whites are racist until proven otherwise—and 'bargainers', such as basketballers Michael Jordan and Magic Johnson, who are loved because they don't embarrass whites by bringing up America's past. Rather than challenge whites, Jordan merely expanded his Airness; that is to say, he dresses smartly, oozes charm instead of perspiration despite using a Hall of Fame speech to trample his enemies and expands his business empire while lowering his golf handicap. Johnson, the first globally famous athlete to contract HIV (via sex with multiple women), could have become an effective anti-AIDS campaigner but, like Jordan, lacked the social conscience of Ali.

Ali belonged to both of Steele's categories, being provocative and loved. The philosopher was also wrong on Obama whom he wrote about in his 2007 book, *A Bound Man: Why We Are Excited About Obama and Why He Can't Win.* Steele calls Obama a 'super-bargainer'—using the term 'Iconic Negro', as he does with

TV host Oprah Winfrey, an influential supporter of the former Chicago senator from the beginning of his campaign.

Australian Aborigines can be similarly pigeonholed in Steele's challengers and bargainers dichotomy. Boxer Anthony Mundine is an obvious challenger, angering many with his post-11 September 2001 remark that the terrorist attacks on New York's Twin Towers were deserved. Like Ali, he also converted to the Muslim religion and frequently evokes white Australia's shameful treatment of indigenous people, particularly the stolen generation. Those who played rugby league with him at St George, before his switch to professional boxing, speak of the two Anthony Mundines: 'the quiet, respectful Choc and the loud, brash Mundine.' Mundine plays off this, knowing there is an uneducated white mob desperate to see him whipped in the ring. He was the only sporting star roundly booed during cricket's Big Bash Victorian Bushfire appeal at the SCG in February 2009, except when he was run out first ball.

Mundine has also upset the more sensitive of the Aboriginal sports stars by demanding they come forward and make similar comments. He sent a verbal straight left to Catherine Freeman, 'Our Cathy' who won Australia's only gold medal on the track at the Sydney Olympics. Freeman has preferred to use her business contacts with an increasing number of female chief executives in banks and the leisure industry to finance her foundation and help the youth of Palm Island, one of the flashpoints of racial tension in Australia. One of the innovative projects involves giving a bike to truants after they demonstrate a regular attendance record at the island's school. The $100,000 payment she received from magazine *New Idea* for exclusive coverage of her second wedding was directed to her foundation.

Cathy prefers to walk this path to assist disadvantaged Aborigines, not simply because she is shy, or lacks confidence speaking in public. She actually enjoys contact with a white, female, upwardly mobile world. I sat with her one night at the Beijing Olympics, on the occasion of the 110-metre men's hurdles final, when China's Liu Xiang was favourite. It had originally loomed as a great story—the woman on whom the hopes of twenty million people had rested in 2000 watching the man carrying the dreams of 1.3 billion people—but Liu withdrew due to injury two days earlier. Freeman asked about Mundine and my knowledge of him via my St George connection. She also reminded me we were both in Victoria, Canada, in 1994, when she ran with the Aboriginal flag after winning the 400-metre final at the Commonwealth Games. I had covered that story for Fairfax and there had been considerable negative reaction to her gesture, principally from Australia's Commonwealth Games chief, Arthur Tunstall. But sitting there in the Bird's Nest stadium in Beijing, Cathy explained to me she felt as much white as black.

'I'm Australian first but I'm also a Pom and happy for their success,' she said of Britain's bulging chest of medals in Beijing and hopes for London 2012. 'The Poms supported me when there was so much controversy in Canada. I spent so much time there. I lived and trained in London and I loved it.' She explained that, while she will always be defined by her essential Australian-ness, her surname—and all it implies—derives from England: 'My great-great-grandfather did come from Dorset,' she said, as grateful for her gifts as her nation is to have her as our own.

The AFL boasts of its disproportionate number of Aboriginal players—four or five times greater representation than in the general population—and the code has certainly produced some men who would fit Steele's 'Iconic Negro' category. Pastor Doug Nicholls, a former tarboy in the shearing sheds, joined Fitzroy and became the first Aboriginal player to represent his state and be knighted. He later became Governor of South Australia. Polly Farmer, formerly of Western Australia, has a gate named after him at the stadium of his club, Geelong. Essendon's Michael Long is much revered and was joined by many whites on his reconciliation march from Melbourne to Canberra.

Long's family are Tiwi Islanders and my wife and I once stayed with their kinsmen, the Riolis, at their island home. They took us to the nearby golf club and its nine 'browns', where the players moved from one hole to the next in a four-wheel-drive vehicle. Michael Long's noble father, clearly the chief of the community, stood on a dusty path watching the play when a herd of water buffalos sauntered out of the bush. I had seen *Crocodile Dundee* hypnotising a giant ox and saw the movie *Australia*, where an Aboriginal lad spooked a herd of prize cattle out of stampeding over a cliff face. And I now witnessed a similar incident firsthand. The lead cattle, emerging from the scrub, took one glance at the sentinel-like Long and did an immediate U-turn back to the safety of the bush. These men all have 'mana'—power, authority, prestige—as the Maoris call it.

Yet my experience with Aboriginal athletes is that they simply want to be treated the same as everyone else in the team. Embracing social causes is perceived to be alienating. I recall a St George lower-grade coach speaking to his players before a match, saying of the opposition, 'There's a few black bastards in their team and you know they can't tackle'. I interjected to say, 'And there's a few white bastards out there as well who can't tackle'. In the hyped pre-game atmosphere, few of the players picked up my unsubtle censure of their coach, but an Aboriginal player did not miss it—his face changed from a mask covering desperately veiled humiliation to relief that the head coach was on his side.

Sometimes a clumsy attempt is made to correct these embarassments, with the coach/manager/fellow player saying, 'I didn't mean you Cedric, you're a white man'. This belongs to the same genre as the post-World War II tuxedoed fight announcers declaring, 'Joe Louis, the heavyweight champion of the world and a credit to his race'. Why should some redneck in black tie be in a position to judge who is a credit and who is not? And, as someone later asked, what race is he talking about? The human race?

The knock on Aboriginal players is that they lack a work ethic on the field; and that they aren't keen on the self-sacrificial tasks, such as head-on tackling, diving on a loose ball, or charging down a kick. They 'go walkabout' when the game grinds to an arm wrestle. Yet could it be just a coincidence that diving for the loose ball is a skill more conveniently executed on the groomed, green fields of private schools than on an outback oval studded with stones, burrs and bare earth? Similarly, in American basketball, some have observed that many of the tasks a player performs in white basketball to prove his character—take charge, scramble for a loose ball—are more pleasantly done on a polished wooden floor than they are on inner-city asphalt. And don't these skills come more readily when the athlete has been educated through a large club or college system?

In any case, aren't blacks supposed to play a different way—to be flashy and score tries and hit baskets? The basketball team, the Harlem Globetrotters, demonstrated this hypocrisy. These stars were paid money to exhibit proof of all the prejudices a white world had created. They were gangling, devious, lazy and did not take the game seriously, being given to outbursts of laughter. Their success depended on slyly outwitting the white referee or white opposition, even inserting a weight inside the bladder of the ball in order for it to bounce at preposterous angles, embarrassing white guards. Yet they had players like 'Wilt' Chamberlain who could beat white professionals at so-called white basketball.

Perhaps it could be argued that their white owner, Abe Saperstein, was doing them a favour—giving them a living in a sport which, in the early days of the professional league, barred them from playing. Yet this comic role-play at the expense of their dignity was used against them when the owner of the Washington Redskins was asked why he didn't have any black players in his NFL team. 'I'll hire blacks when I see whites playing for the Harlem Globetrotters', was the essence of his reply. When black players finally did make it into the NBA, the rule was: 'You start two blacks at home, three on the road and five when you're 18 points behind.' Now, 85 per cent of players in the NBA are African-American.

On the other hand, the number of black baseballers is declining rapidly, coincidentally with the rise of the Latino player. One of the reasons—an accusation levelled by former black ballplayers against recently retired African-American superstars—is they don't put anything back into the communities which produced them. They detach themselves and return no social good to their roots, which are left worse than before. They often end up with little of their wealth.

The AFL has been hypocritical in its so-called enlightened attitude to Aboriginal players. In 1987, alarmed by an eleven per cent fall in attendance, the AFL commissioned an advertising campaign that focused on the Krakouer brothers and their 'black magic'. The campaign probably embarrassed the brothers because it separated them from their team mates and may have offended rednecks who saw Aborigines in the unaccustomed position of being in charge, even if it was just on a football field. Jimmy Krakouer was sledged relentlessly and retaliated, losing 22 games to suspension.

Then followed Nicky Winmar's famous gesture in 1993 at Collingwood's then home ground of Victoria Park, when he pulled up his jumper and pointed to his stomach. It was widely interpreted that Winmar was pointing to his skin—an 'up yours' to a racist section of the Collingwood crowd who had been heckling the St Kilda player throughout the match. The AFL has allowed a degree of historical revisionism to travel in tandem with this incident and the subsequent success of its anti-racial vilification campaign. Yet some of Winmar's team mates within earshot, and Winmar himself, have told commentators that he was referring not to his skin but his guts. He was pointing out that, unlike the hecklers hiding on a hill of anonymity, he had the fortitude to get out on the field and perform.

The reality is the Winmar incident did not launch the AFL's anti-vilification campaign. This came two years later when one of the AFL's most prominent officials, Collingwood president, Allan McAlister, made the stupid comment about Aborigines being treated the same as whites, provided they behave like them. And one of his players, Damian Monkhorst, called Long a 'black cunt'. The AFL, embarrassed by the comments of the president of its most popular club and the disrespect to Long, finally decided to act.

The rugby codes never felt the need to trumpet their Aboriginal players until the AFL's widely promoted 'indigenous round' forced the NRL to act. A team of Indigenous All Stars was chosen by public vote to play a February 2010 game against a team of NRL All Stars. Aboriginal players like Mark Ella and Arthur Beetson have captained the Wallabies and Kangaroos respectively, while Mal Meninga, who considers himself of Pacific Island heritage, has also skippered Australia. Beetson and Meninga were both chosen in rugby league's Team of the Century. However, another Team of the Century member, halfback Andrew Johns, undid much of rugby league's good work in promoting the role of Indigenous players when he made a racist comment while in camp as an assistant coach with the NSW State of Origin team in June 2010. Johns made derogatory remarks about Queensland's preponderance of Aboriginal and Polynesian players in an antediluvian attempt to inspire the predominatly white Blues. A NSW Aboriginal player, Tamana Taahua, who was also a former team mate of Johns', walked out of the camp in protest and Johns resigned his post.

Today, both rugby codes struggle to accommodate the surging number of players from Polynesian backgrounds and a diverse culture that ranges from church-going, teetotalling Tongans to party-loving Maoris.

Forty per cent of NRL players are of Polynesian or indigenous heritage but over a half of the code's elite under-20 league and two-thirds of junior representative teams from western Sydney are of Polynesian descent. Polynesian players are called 'freshies' by their team mates, as in 'fresh off the boat', having spent a couple of years in New Zealand before trialling for an NRL contract. The next generation of talent, however, is Australian born and seeking the traditional path to the top via the code's established elite junior pathways.

The Polynesian player is the elephant in the rugby league dressing room. Officials, fearful of being accused of racism, won't comment about his impact in the junior leagues, where he stampedes over lighter and whiter opponents, or the challenge he represents to the entrenched ethos of some traditional NRL clubs who simply don't know how to deal with these players. Nor do the Polynesian players seek any political influence in the dressing room. Most NRL clubs have a leadership group elected by the players and Polynesian numbers are such that they could easily combine to vote one of their own on, yet they don't do so. They refuse to use sport to advance a social cause.

Stephen Kearney, assistant coach of the Storm and head coach of the winning World Cup New Zealand team, says the answer is simple. 'The island boys and the Maoris are like anyone, including the Aboriginal lads', says Kearney, a Maori. 'They just want to be seen to be the same as everyone else, while retaining their cultural identity which means a lot.' Asked why some are devoutly religious and others enjoy a night on the tiles, Kearney observes, 'Put it down to Captain Cook discovering New Zealand before the missionaries found Tonga and Samoa.'

Golfer Tiger Woods, like Cathy Freeman, is another sports star whom militant blacks say has pressed the mute button on his social conscience. He's perceived to be black but as his mother, Tida, says, he is a racial bouillabaisse. 'Tiger has Thai, African, Chinese, American-Indian and European blood', she once said. 'He is the Universal Child.' Perhaps it's best to think of him as having the best of all the bloodlines. Tiger's rise in a sport that was once considered to be the preserve of wealthy whites to the lofty position of top earner in all sports is phenomenal. At the peak of his power, he earned twice the next highest paid and nearly three times the third.

Tiger's rise may well have been independent of a social revolution on American golf courses, which began with an interview in 1990 by a general assignment reporter for the *Birmingham Post-Herald*, subsequently reported by the world's best sports magazine, *Sports Illustrated*. The reporter sat down with Hall Thompson, the founder of a private golf club at nearby Shoal Creek, the site of the PGA Championship that year. During the interview, the then 67-year-old Thompson, a wealthy businessman, uttered the unpardonable words that probably made him Alabama's second most-significant catalyst for change in US race relations. (No. 1 will always be Rosa Parks, the African-American seamstress who ignited the civil rights movement when she refused to offer her seat on a Montgomery bus to a white man in 1955.) Thompson told the reporter in response to a question about Shoal Creek excluding blacks from membership: 'Bringing up this issue will just polarise the community . . . but it can't pressure us . . . We have the right to associate or not to associate with whomever we choose. The country club is our home and we pick and choose who we want . . . I think we've said we don't discriminate in every other area except the blacks.'

Thompson's answer opened a cellar door to expose the worst-kept secret in golf—the undeniable whiteness of the game in the United States. Surprisingly, there was no major civil rights protest and Jim Thorpe, then the only African-American on the tour qualifiers that year, said of a possible boycott, 'I've got a family to feed.' Only Lee Elder, the first black golfer to play in the US Masters, showed any glimmer of social conscience when he said of Shoal Creek's limp compensatory offer of an honorary membership to a black Birmingham businessman, 'An honorary membership doesn't mean anything.'

But the PGA Tour took action. It announced it would not hold tournaments on courses that discriminated on the basis of race, religion, sex or national origin. Even the elitist Augusta National, home of the Masters, surrendered its plantation mentality, adding a black member, the first since Bobby Jones founded the club in 1932. The PGA Tour action was swift, considering the relatively mute press and protest. Ironically, American business forced the revolution. Computer giant IBM had refused to advertise on ABC's telecast of the Shoal Creek tournament and this started a stampede of sponsors running away. In other words, the same American businessmen distancing themselves from the exclusionary practices of private clubs were the same businessmen who institutionalised the racist, sexist and chauvinistic structure of these clubs.

Compounding the irony was that these events precipitated a Great White Hunt for blacks to join these clubs—men previously barred because of the pigmentation of their skin were now being sought for the same wrong reason. One high-profile black approached to join a club with a Nicklaus-designed course near Los Angeles was O.J. Simpson, the former NFL star and endorser of a range of American products. Simpson overlooked the obvious hypocrisy and accepted the invitation, saying, 'I expect this whole Shoal Creek incident will be remembered some day almost like the Boston Tea Party. Ten years, a hundred years from now, when we see mixed golf everywhere, we'll remember this as one of the single most important incidents in our history.'

These thoughts were expressed a few years before O.J. was charged with the double murder of his estranged wife and her lover. Interestingly, I was in Boston in October 1995 when his 'not guilty' verdict was handed down in a national broadcast. It was lunchtime and my wife and I were in a bar with maybe a hundred people, only half a dozen of whom were black, all hanging on the result of one of the most discussed trials in US history. The verdict was received with stunned silence by the whites—bar some muttering—but there was wild, provocative cheering by the small group of blacks. It wasn't the type of integration that O.J. had predicted would come from the Shoal Creek incident, but then O.J. won't be remembered how he would like to be.

The reality is that Tiger Woods probably did as much for black golfers as Shoal Creek. In July 1990, in the midst of the Shoal Creek affair, *Sports Illustrated* asked: 'Who will be the next black trailblazer on the Tour?' 'The most likely candidate is 14-year-old Eldrick (Tiger) Woods of Cypress, California. Tiger is a +2 handicapper who has already won four junior world championships—more than Mark O'Meara or Craig Stadler did as kids . . . he probably won't be a regular on the Tour until the year 2000.'

Even *Sports Illustrated* did not foresee the phenomenal rise of Tiger. By 2000, he had not only overwhelmed his sport, he had re-arranged it, making even the most accomplished rivals appear uncomfortable and unworthy. He was No. 1 golfer in the world and had won all four majors. In 2000 alone, he wrought the greatest season in golf history, winning ten tournaments, including three majors. The one that eluded him—the Masters—he had already won in 1997 by a margin of twelve strokes. In that tournament, he drove the ball so far with his prodigious physical gifts, it appeared as if he was playing a shorter, easier course than his rivals.

By 2000, the four major championships had been played 344 times and Tiger owned, or co-owned, the scoring record in all four and was the youngest—by two years—to do so. But the naysayers argued he hadn't won a Grand Slam because his victories in the four majors weren't achieved in the same calendar year. The critics went back 50 years to find Ben Hogan, who won a hat trick in 1953; Bobby Jones won a Grand Slam in 1930 and in 1945; Byron Nelson won eighteen tournaments, including eleven consecutively.

But Jones' Grand Slam was vastly different to the modern version. He won the US and the British Opens but they were amateur events—meaning he didn't have to face the era's top professionals. Nelson's epic year came when the world was at war; he won the only major played in 1945 (the PGA) but to be fair, one of the golfers missing was Captain Ben Hogan of the US Army Air Corp, not discharged until after the war. Eight years later, in Hogan's signature season, he won his three majors by a combined fifteen strokes, which was Woods' margin of victory at the 2000 US Open.

So, just as everyone was debating what constituted a Grand Slam—four consecutive opens, or four in a calendar year—Tiger did all that was available to him. He won the next Masters, in April 2001, by two strokes, completing the sweep—the first man ever to win four majors in a row. It was only four years after he turned pro and last won the Masters, the first black man ever to win at snow-white Augusta.

Even then, as the new century dawned, critics argued the competition wasn't as strong as in say Jack Nicklaus' day. Yet David Duval's 14-under par 274 in the 2001 Masters would have won 59 of the 65 Masters ever played and sent him into a playoff in another two. In fact, some quipped that the golfers born around the same time as Tiger belong to an Unlucky Procreation Club.

If you look at another yardstick by which golfers are measured—prize money—Tiger's earnings were more than twice the next man. And if money is an inappropriate topic of conversation in the clubhouse, his number of ranking points was double the next.

Muhammad Ali was great but was he twice as good as Joe Frazier? Don Bradman was twice as good as the next batsmen in terms of batting average, but he did have team mates—he couldn't control the game on his own. Okay, Michael Jordan had team mates and beat opponents one on two, but he wasn't twice as good as Magic Johnson or Larry Bird. Tiger was alone. Nobody of his calibre has ever been on the same fairway.

When he won his second Masters, he carried the entire world of golf on his back. He won the 2008 US Open on one leg, a feat which didn't surprise those who believed he walked on water. When he returned to the course nine months after a knee reconstruction, he won a tournament simply by putting. But in the 2009 PGA, he led into the final round and lost to a Korean, Y.E. Yang. It was the first time he had ever lost a major after leading the tournament entering the final day and, coincidentally, the first win by an Asian-born golfer. Nicklaus has more Grand Slams—eighteen to Tiger's fourteen. Nicklaus had nineteen seconds in majors but Tiger has never appeared interested in being, as comedian Jerry Seinfeld describes second place, 'the No. 1 loser'.

And TV—the nervous medium that forced the Shoal Creek revolution—loves him. When he teed off in the 2000 US Open with a ten-stroke lead on the final day—virtually six hours of exhibition golf ahead—NBC's ratings were eleven per cent up on the previous year. He not only lived up to our expectations, he bettered our impossible dreams. No wonder his visit to Melbourne to play in the November 2009 Masters—for a take-home fee of $3 million courtesy of the Victorian taxpayer—attracted huge galleries, and caused traffic jams and helicopters to hover overhead during Tiger's practice round. The event generated massive publicity for Melbourne and Tiger went along with it, presenting himself as equal parts cliché and politeness.

Not known at the time was Tiger was in a very bad lie. He was sleeping with a woman flown to Australia by his management and he was also gambling heavily at Melbourne's Crown Casino. A week later—just when the world believed Tiger's only competition was with himself and Nicklaus' legacy—he was forced to quit golf indefinitely. An early morning altercation with his Swedish born wife, Elin, led to him crashing his car on the driveway of his Florida mansion and the rapid unravelling of what was perceived to be a perfect family life. The matrimonial argument involved his infidelity and, as more than a dozen women claimed to have had affairs with him, the joke circulated Tiger was now 'playing on the back nine'.

Sponsors deserted him, particularly those who had used him as the smiling face of their global marketing campaigns. Gatorade, the sports drink company, was first out, and then TAG Heuer, makers of prestige watches, quickly followed. Gillette, always conscious of its clean-cut image, had only weeks earlier endured bad publicity when another of their corporate totems—French soccer captain Thierry Henry—allowed his handball to force Ireland out of the 2010 World Cup. Irishmen swore never to shave and Gillette now found itself running into further stubble with Tiger, their smiling beacon in sunglasses. Gillette pulled the plug, leaving Nike as Tiger's main backer.

Nike Golf, whose total sales of US$600 million in 2007 were largely inspired by Tiger's pitch, would always be the last to sack him. Nike has always been closely identified with status, glamour, being cool and competitive. The swoosh emblem is a tick for living on the edge, as Tiger had been doing clandestinely for years, chasing tail. Traditionally, Nike has always valued iconoclasts with big-time attitudes, more than being interested in investing in grassroots sport. Nike executives have courted athletes like tennis players Andre Agassi, John McEnroe and Ilie Năstase, and American footballers and basketballers of the type who embarrass grown-ups. Its corporate imperatives mock the perceived values manufacturers of sports products sanctimoniously claim to be protecting, such as respect for their opponent and fair play. Nike has therefore been a lightning rod for the increased ambivalence people feel about the convergence of sport and business and the extent to which risk-taking has become a glamorous end in itself.

Nike executives, as well as the management team of Tiger Inc., probably turned a blind eye to his liaisons with a string of cocktail waitresses, nightclub hostesses and porn actresses. Golf writers, too, would have been aware of his philandering, in the same way his fellow players would have pretended not to see. But if TV ratings are any guide, golf without Tiger is a tropical beach without sunsets. Why rat on the man who is responsible for your newspaper flying you around the world, or risk the opprobrium of your fellow writers to out Tiger? If you are a player, why jeopardise your appearance money? Significantly, the only professional golfer who demonised Woods after the revelations of his infidelity was the obscure Swedish golfer who introduced Tiger to his future wife, Elin. Tiger's first public appearance after his ignominy was a stage-managed press conference. After a month of sex therapy, he admitted he needed to restore his old values. 'I need to go back to my old roots,' he said—words that drew a chuckle in Australia.

He chose the US Masters in Augusta for his return; an unfortunate choice because the club excludes women as members. But Augusta—the Cathedral of golf—could guarantee Tiger wouldn't be heckled and the galleries treated him kindly. It's interesting to reflect what that old cynic, Oscar Wilde, would have made of it. The nineteenth-century Irish poet once observed, 'The Americans are certainly hero-worshippers and always take their heroes from the criminal classes.' Tiger didn't commit a crime, but after a month in a sex clinic where he was treated for an addiction, he may have felt he did. Oscar could have been talking equally about Australia and our hero-worshipping of Ned Kelly. Certainly, in the audience at Augusta were representatives of Victorian Major Events, desperate to convince Tiger's management he was welcome back in Melbourne.

Annika Sörenstam, also sits in the golf pantheon with Tiger. Tiger's 2002 record—when he won only six of 22 starts—compares dismally with Sweden's Ice Queen. In that same year, she won more than half her starts—thirteen of 25 tournaments around the world. 'If Tiger had a year like Annika,' complained LPGA player Jill McGill, 'they'd reschedule sunsets for him.' Still, American golfer Michelle Wie—tipped as a twelve year old to become women golf's Tiger—took eight years of trying before she won a professional tournament. Wie's shot-making has long amazed many male viewers. Born of South Korean parents, she was more accomplished at thirteen than the male golfing Mozart, Tiger Woods. She was the youngest person ever to win a USPGA event in which adults compete. Just as Tiger and Pinocchio were turned on the lathes of their father's ambitions, so was this 68-kilogram teen who can blast tee shots 30 yards (27.43 metres) farther than battle-hardened LPGA pros—and even a handful of PGA Tour players. However, after winning the US Women's Public Links title as a thirteen year old, she was winless on the LPGA tour until she finally broke through in 2009. She said of her post-victory celebrations: 'Just seeing them come out and pour beer all over me, it was a great feeling. I've always seen it on TV, and I've always wanted people to pour beer on me.'

In terms of the big picture, the sports world seems to classify women as either disposable or as a nuisance. Women's sport does not attract the ratings, gates, sponsorship or media space of male sport. The only area where it wins is government grants.

The biggest press conference I ever attended concerned a sports star who didn't turn up and the athlete in question wasn't a male. During the lead-up to the February 1994 Winter Olympics in Lillehammer, Norway, there had been growing rumours US ice-skater, Tonya Harding, was implicated in a plot to destroy the chances of her main rival for an Olympic gold medal, compatriot Nancy Kerrigan. Kerrigan was clubbed above the right knee by a goon carrying an iron bar at a practice session held during the US National Figure Skating Championships in Detroit the previous month. Harding and Kerrigan had entered the winter season as leading contenders for a gold medal, with a possible $10 million payout in endorsements, appearance and tours for the Olympic champion. It was a tangled story of thuggery, sex, lies, athletic ambition and financial gain, played out against the backdrop of a Games held in a pure-white snow kingdom straight out of a Hansel and Gretel world.

With Kerrigan injured, Harding won the event in Detroit. But a few days later, Harding's ex-husband, Jeff Gillooly, and her bodyguard admitted hiring the goon who attacked Kerrigan. As part of a plea bargain, Gillooly revealed Harding approved the plot.

When the US Figure Skating Association and the US Olympic Committee initiated proceedings against Harding to ban her from competing in Lillehammer, Harding threatened legal action and retained her place on the US team. Kerrigan was also selected for Lillehammer.

Harding arrived in Norway to the type of reception usually reserved for the monarch, King Harald V. She appeared on the cover of both *Time* and *Newsweek*. At Hammer airport, so frenetic were the media struggles to woo a word, seek a smile, line-up a lens on the ice maiden from Portland, Oregon, that the Norwegian Minister for Agriculture, who happened to be in the neighbourhood, was elbowed out of the way. Through it all, Harding smiled sweetly, saying, 'Thanks for coming guys. I'm going to win. I feel great. I'm ready.' Each word was recorded like holy writ.

As if Harding's presence and the publicity surrounding her were not embarrassing enough to Olympic officials, her arrival had been preceded by the publication in a London tabloid of a display of photographs of her topless. The photos had been taken from a pornographic video, entitled 'Wedding Video', where Harding was filmed having sex with Gillooly. There was talk of a possible *Penthouse* centrefold. She had been warned by the USFSA not to 'play any tricks', including any attempt to proceed with her widely quoted desire to hug Kerrigan. More than 700 journalists and photographers watched Harding and Kerrigan skate at practice and over 1200 attended a Kerrigan press conference, more than heard Carl Lewis speak after his gold medal haul at the 1984 Los Angeles Olympics.

But the biggest press contingent attended the conference where Harding's coach, Diane Rawlinson, was expected to shed some light on Gillooly's claim Harding was involved in the attack on

Kerrigan. Rawlinson, dressed in a hand-knitted white woollen jumper featuring cuddly animals, spoke only of God and Harding's focus. She even converted focus to an adjective, saying, 'Figure skating is a very focal sport.' Journalists seeking to gain more information for the good-queen Kerrigan–evil-queen Harding story, left disappointed. As events transpired, neither American skater won the gold medal, which went to Ukraine's Oksana Baiul. Harding ended the Games hanging out with the male bobsledders, drinking shots and playing pool.

A week after the Lillehammer Olympics, Harding entered a plea bargain to avoid prison, admitting complicity in the Kerrigan attack and, on 30 June, she was stripped of her 1994 national title and banned for life from the sport. She was also not admitted to the professional ranks, meaning she never benefitted from the pro tour boom that ensued in the aftermath of the scandal she helped create. She took up boxing and won a bout on the undercard to a Mike Tyson fight. A match-up with Daisy Do, a transvestite at a Fort Lauderdale bar was cancelled because the Florida Boxing Commission refused to sanction it.

It seems to me the biggest stories in female sport concern women behaving badly. Women's soccer is very big in the United States, but some of the most popular internet video hits concerned a college defender pulling down her opponent by her ponytail and also a late game brawl between high school girls. Men have a curious fascination with females fighting and the 2009 online shots of women players punching, kicking and scratching rivals attracted as many viewers as the US women's win in the World Cup.

Dawn Fraser is Australia's most famous female sports figure, not perhaps because she won gold medals in the same event at three successive Olympics but because she has been an enduring larrikin—stealing a Japanese flag at the Tokyo Olympics and banned from competition for life; having a covert relationship with a top rugby league player; flirting with lesbianism; entering state politics as an independent; and even, at age 71, claiming to capture an intruder at her Noosa home.

One of the most explosive stories in Australian sport came at the 2004 Athens Olympics when a rower in the women's eight, Sally Robbins, stopped rowing during the race, earning the nickname, 'Lay Down Sally'. She expressed no remorse at the post-race media conference, focusing on her own performance rather than expressing any sympathy to her team mates. A midnight mediation session involving former Wallaby captain John Eales—an athlete liaison officer with the Australian team in Athens—did not resolve the matter. One rower, Catriona Oliver, slapped Robbins at an Olympic team function in Sydney and was given a two-year suspended sentence. Parents of the crew sought counselling and dredged up earlier examples of Robbins' collapses in races, blaming coaches for selecting her for Athens. The ripples of the affair extended to other sports, including the Parramatta rugby league team where it became a case study in team disintegration. AOC president John Coates won a big defamation payment from broadcaster Alan Jones who had claimed Coates instructed the rowers on what to say at their press conference.

At popular international events, such as the Olympics, Commonwealth Games and World Championships, women attract equal publicity, create mountains of goodwill and achieve a level of celebrity. Then, with the Games over, they recede from the public consciousness. Australia's female swimmers, such as Susie O'Neill and Samantha Rice, generate the same TV ratings as men at World Championships but they stay on in the headlines only via celebrity publicity, such as Rice's romantic interests and post-Olympics partying. Yet Australia's female gold-medal-winning Olympians—such as Fraser, Betty Cuthbert, Marjorie Jackson through to Winter Games winners such as Alisa Camplin and Lydia Lassila—have carried the nation in terms of medal success over the past hundred years.

If male officials have let their athletes down, the bosses of women's sports have been worse. When women's sports administrators vent their complaints, they talk problems and rarely solutions. They are only too willing to discuss the reasons why the male sports world is rife with bad boys, while their girls are wonderful role models. Their long list of laments include the inflated salaries of male sports stars and their expectation of entitlement, the male's life of pampering since high school, the innate gender differences and an old boys' media network that tolerates anti-social behaviour from male athletes. The notion of women athletes engaging in behaviour such as group sex and communal drug-taking is ludicrous but this does not excuse women's sport bosses for hectoring males about such inequities. I recall appearing before a Senate enquiry into women's sport and seemingly being held personally responsible for limited coverage in *The Sydney Morning Herald*. When I mentioned that many of the *SMH* pages are given over to covering 'neutral' events, such as horseracing, I was lampooned for suggesting women were interested in the gallops. This was, admittedly, before the ascent of trainer Gai Waterhouse and jockey Michelle Payne.

Female officials should remember that netball or women's cricket is a sport, not a cause. The athletes are over the the banner-carrying phase but their leaders are not. Most female athletes are engaging and cooperative and have a sense of humour. One of my colleagues justified the 1990s ban on female journalists entering the Balmain rugby league dressing room on the basis that male journalists could not enter a netball change room. The netballer, Liz Ellis, listening to the argument, used it to point to her sport's antiquated facilities: 'You can interview me but it will have to be on the back seat of my car', she said, clearly implying this is where she dressed for games.

The ABC was the only TV network to cover the Australia versus England women's cricket test in Perth, held as part of the celebrations of Victoria's sesquicentenary. Two male commentators, the late Wally Foreman and Dennis Cometti, had a private bet that whoever was called upon to interview the English captain during the lunch break would ask her if she wore protective clothing. With Cometti doing the interview and the floor manager winding it to a close, Foreman began congratulating himself on winning the bet. But Cometti made it his final question. 'Do you wear a box?' he asked. 'Yes, we do Dennis', the English captain replied gracefully. 'Except we call it a man-hole cover.'

Women's sport officials are always more serious. They rarely consider marketing to both genders. Most of their paid spectators are likely to be either family or women and girls, but men make up most of the couch potato demographic that drives TV ratings. Nor do women's sport administrators have patience in the demand for equality with men. Male sports have been accumulating fans and history for decades.

Women administrators take disparate views on using sex to promote their sports, some confusing selling sex appeal with selling sex. Netball officials haven't shown any ambivalence. Thirty years ago, they ordered their athletes out of box tunics and dressed them in short skirts. Australian golfer Jan Stephenson oozed sex appeal and sold her sport, an effective counter to those who dub women golfers 'dykes on spikes.' Women's beach volleyball pulls big crowds at the Olympics because the athletes are dressed in bikinis and they are in super physical shape. The serves and returns of women's beach volleyball players are in the same park as the baggy-short wearing men, usually recruited from those who have failed to make the cut as footballers or athletes in other Olympic sports. The TV ratings of women's hockey at the Olympics are similar to men's, because whatever superior skills sets the men possess, it is balanced by the athleticism and attractiveness of the Hockeyroos.

Sex without skills does not work. Tennis player Anna Kournikova made plenty of money and looked hot pulling the second ball from under the lining of her knickers but she did not advance her sport. She didn't win a tournament and was lampooned as Anna 'Pornikova.' Her Slavic successors are comfortable being both strong, winning athletes and alluring, sexually attractive celebrities.

But a sport that rejects sex appeal and is a weaker, less skilful version of the male game will never attract crowds or TV ratings. Exhibit A: women's cricket. Its players are clothed in white (although often not in dresses these days) but, because it is a less spectacularly skilful game than the male equivalent, its Test matches are played in provincial towns, or obscure grounds like Drummoyne Oval.

On the other hand, some male-dominated sports will never accept women as anything more than tokens. This was evidenced in the words of Formula 1 chief Bernie Ecclestone when asked whether he would endorse a woman driver. 'I don't care who drives,' he said, and then added, clearly seeking someone who ticked all the minority boxes, 'It would be fantastic to have a female pilot who is black and Jewish.'

Nor have the achievements of many women athletes been given due credit. In 2002, English athlete Paula Radcliffe ran a marathon in two hours and seventeen minutes, not only shattering the women's world record but narrowing to twelve minutes the gap between the men's and women's best times. It meant that in the previous 40 years, women had improved their record by more than an hour and men by nine minutes. People finally came to the view women had a superior build to men for marathon running, a far cry from the days they were warned not to run because their uteruses might fall out.

Male comedians have long told 'gender bender' gags, such as the two leading British female Olympians who might possibly have less clearance over the hurdles than other women in the same race. And there were multiple snickers when it was revealed 'Stella was a fella'—the gold-medal-winning athlete at the 1932 Los Angeles Olympics, Stella Walsh, was murdered during a 1980 bottle shop robbery and when doctors performed an autopsy they discovered she was male. Walsh also won a silver medal at the 1936 Berlin Olympics, at the same stadium which was the scene of another gender case in August 2009.

The Caster Semenya story demonstrated that track-and-field officials haven't learnt much in the 30 years since Walsh died. Semenya, a South African eighteen-year-old middle distance runner, won the women's 800-metre title at the 2009 World Championships in Berlin; yet, even before the race, there were reports she was male. Her musculature, running style and recent stunning improvement in times suggested she was male. South African track-and-field officials initially denied any gender tests were done of Semenya before the team left South Africa but later admitted to lying to protect her. Semenya had been taken to a hospital in Pretoria where her feet were put in stirrups and photographs were taken of her genitalia during a two-hour examination. She had been told the tests were done for doping reasons. The South African team doctor informed his country's top athletics officials that Semenya should not compete but they ignored the advice, allowing her to travel to Germany. Basically, she was humiliated in order for South Africa to win a gold medal.

The IOC responded to the case by announcing its Medical Commission would organise a symposium to examine the gender issue and advise sports bodies how to respond. Admittedly, the Semenya case was one of the most challenging in the Orwellian arena of 'gender verification' because, externally, she appeared to be female, yet internally had male reproductive organs. IOC Medical Commission chairman Arne Ljungqvist alluded to this hermaphroditism, saying, 'Sometimes you come across cases that are uncertain and ambiguous, and it changes from being a sports matter to a medical matter. That's where we need to have a review.' However, the 'where' the review took place is interesting: Florida, in January 2010—just the place to visit in the midst of the northern hemisphere winter.

In Australia, the reality is women's sport has been heavily funded by government in order for it to receive any prominence. When Prime Minister Malcolm Fraser was booed by Australian Olympians during a visit to the athletes village in Montreal in 1976, he was so embarrassed he ordered his ministers to dust off a report on a sports institute commissioned by the Whitlam Government. Australia did not collect a single gold medal in Montreal but by

Seoul in 1988, the results of Canberra's Australian Institute of Sport were evident, with golds won by the Hockeyroos and by Debbie Flintoff's victory in the 400-metre hurdles.

The ASC—the sports funding arm of the federal government set up in 1984 by the Hawke Government—paid for the production costs when the ABC began providing coverage of netball. This was a time when TV's answer to most women's sport was the reverse of the old commercial for women's tennis . . . Sorry, baby, you haven't come a long way. When the ABC dumped netball and Fox Sport began televising the trans-Tasman league, the federal government again tipped in with a heavy subsidy. Netball is now on free-to-air commercial TV and Australian governments of both political persuasions are committed to correcting the gender imbalance, with the Rudd Government directing that half its $32 million windfall to soccer go to further development of teams in a women's league.

Men Are from Mars, Women Are from Venus when it comes to coaching. The classic example of the difference is how males and females respond when a coach berates a team. If a coach tells a women's team that some players aren't pulling their weight, every player will duck her head and think the coach is referring to her. If a coach tells a male team the same thing, most men will assume, 'At least he doesn't mean me'. Yet even boys from an early age understand that sport creates hierarchies and the ball must go to the best player whenever he calls for it. Girls must assess you first: they must decide whether they like you before they let you into their circle.

Women are simultaneously more sensitive and more demanding of each other, a lethal combination for a coach seeking the correct team chemistry. The most successful coach in US women's soccer was a male, Anson Dorrance, the legendary coach of the North Carolina university team, known as the Tar Heels. He had a sign in his office which read: 'PEOPLE DON'T CARE HOW MUCH YOU KNOW UNTIL THEY KNOW HOW MUCH YOU CARE.' In other words, 'You can't get me to do anything, unless you care about me first'. Men, on the other hand, are more pragmatic; they seek knowledge that will help them win games and retain their place in the team.

The difference between men and women, according to Dorrance, is evidenced when they arrive for training. The girls slowly put on their shoes, form into groups of two and three, stretch slowly, jog off out of earshot of the coach and catch up on what they have been doing since the last training session. They are socialising. Men chide latecomers and basically want the whole session over as quickly as possible. They will only stall the start of training if rain threatens a series of 400-metre sprints, or some other drill they loathe.

The Australian women's Olympic gold-medal-winning water polo team in Sydney 2000 were proactive in resolving their problems, reaching an unusual agreement with their Hungarian male coach. Aware they might provoke him if they challenged him openly, they had him agree to an arrangement whereby one of their trusted advisers—the principal scientist at the NSW Institute of Sport—would hear all their grievances and then report them anonymously to the coach.

Curiously, some of the best male coaches of women's teams have been accused of sexual assault, as was Dorrance. Many of these accusations have come as a major shock to other female members of the team. When one of Queensland's most successful swim coaches was accused of sexual assault, one of his best, most decent and honest squad members—Olympic gold medallist Susie O'Neill—had no knowledge of any relationship or rancour between the coach and the accusing athlete. Inevitably, such episodes raise the question of whether there is sexual harassment or disappointment? But the alternative—women coaching women—doesn't necessarily work. 'Women coaches can dig too deep', one prominent female athlete has said. 'They want a reason for everything.'

Raelene Boyle, one of Australia's best 200-metre runners, had a difficult relationship with her coach, Shirley Strickland, who was herself an Olympic medal winner. 'Her last words to me in Montreal were, "Whatever you do, don't break",' Raelene once told me. 'So what did I do with that thought flooding through my mind? Break!'

Strickland was a wonderful pioneer for women in the workplace. A brilliant scientist, she was barred from entering one university faculty because they didn't have a women's toilet in the building. But she directed most of her venom against women. I recall Australia's Helsinki Olympic sprinter, John Treloar, telling me about a car journey back from an inner-west Sydney reunion of the 1952 team. He drove Strickland and Marjorie Jackson, then Governor of South Australia, to their city hotel. 'They were sitting together in the back seat and Shirl did not say a word to Marj', a disappointed Treloar recalled.

Yet women can support each other through sport in ways men would find impossible, even unnecessary. An historian, Nikki Henningham, gave a Melbourne University conference on 'Cultural Differences in Sport', fascinating insights into our past, hitherto unreported. She told of the formation in Sydney at the end of World War I of the City Girls' Amateur Sports Association, as a way of enhancing women's potential as leaders and citizens. It ended with the Depression. She also told of Ronda Kimble, who was for 50 years a netball umpire and started netball clubs and competitions in the 1960s. Ronda did fit her wedding day around matches but husbands usually intervened, insisting their wives not train until the household chores were completed. One nasty fellow overloaded his wife with chores that weren't finished until 10.30 pm. Her team mates, rather than cause an embarrassment by marching to the house and helping her with the chores, would simply wait at training until she arrived.

Homosexuality—or, perhaps, more commonly, bisexuality—has been a bigger issue in women's sport than men's. Lesbian relationships tend to be more open, more enduring and, at the top level of sport, more widespread than male gay relationships. In the early days of tennis—as in golf today—it was a matter of intense and immediate speculation among the athletes as to whether new tourcomers were gay or straight. In fact, to fend off the advances of sexual predators of both genders, some women tennis players felt the need to rush into marriages that were foredoomed to failure.

As evidence is increasingly presented that people are born with homosexual predispositions, it is argued that 'masculine' females gravitate to stereotypical 'male' activities, because that's where their talents lie. In other words, they become involved in sport from an early age. Yet even before the growing evidence of a link between heredity and sexual preference, coaches from the old Communist bloc attributed their success with female Olympians to recruiting women of 'masculine' orientation. This was despite the greater stigma homosexuality has in Eastern Europe.

Women track athletes claim lesbianism is not significant in their sport but they don't deny occasional bisexuality, which they attribute to being so physical and in tune with their bodies—a kind of kinship of the senses. Women's sports administrators are reluctant to address lesbianism or bisexuality, yet it can be a legitimate source of enquiry into what makes great athletes tick, just as a study of diet, exercise physiology or sports science can be. Perhaps they are avoiding the inconvenient truth as they seek to dispel the notion that women who excel in sport tend to be unfeminine.

While women's hockey understandably did nothing when its best player left Australia to live with the captain of Holland's women's team, other sports have been almost confrontational in rejecting a lesbian connection. Netball in its early days dressed their stars in slinky black gowns, potentially antagonising a section of the support base. Some call this the 'hyperhetero-sexualisation' of women's sports—a form of homophobia where administrators emphasise traditional femininity because the advertisers and TV networks, which wield power, will find it more palatable.

Former rugby league international, Ian Roberts, is the only footballer in Australia to come out while actually still playing, suggesting many male homosexual athletes avoid confrontation or fear a commercial backlash. Roberts was almost immediately accepted by his peers, despite one North Sydney front-rower—frightened of AIDS—telling the referee when a bloodied Roberts was about to pack into a scrum, 'Put the poof in the second row'. Yet even the most antediluvian of us can become enlightened, admittedly if money is involved. Rugby league immortal, Graeme Langlands, helped design a pair of leggings for athletes, marketed as 'skins', or 'tights'. When Beijing gold-medal diver, Matthew Mitcham, a prominent gay, endorsed a pair of these leggings,

'Changa' told me, 'I'm just dirty Matthew didn't wear the tights when he led the Mardi Gras parade'. Gareth Thomas, the most capped Wales international with 100 rugby tests, as well as being a former British and Irish Lions captain, said when he finally came out, 'I was like a ticking time bomb. I thought I could suppress it, keep it locked away in some dark corner of myself . . . ' Thomas subsequently switched codes and joined a Welsh rugby league team, the Crusaders, further demonstrating that the 13-a-side game is not as neanderthal as the bow-tied essayists think.

One of the most thoughtful athletes I have ever interviewed was George Foreman, the African-American who became the oldest heavyweight champion of the world. Foreman was in Melbourne for the 2006 Commonwealth Games when I met him. He was counterculture in so many ways. His most cherished memory was winning a gold medal in Mexico City in 1968, a time when black sociology professors in the United States were calling for a boycott of the Games, claiming blacks were being used to bring international acclaim to a nation that spurned them at home. 'When I was standing on that platform at age nineteen with the gold medal around my neck, dressed in the American uniform, the national anthem playing and no police chasing me . . . nothing I have done in sport has topped that', he told me.

Foreman draped himself in patriotism, waving the American flag, attracting criticism because it was perceived to be an act of defiance against his fellow Americans, Tommy Smith and John Carlos, who used the podium after the 200-metre final to make their Black Power salute, clenching their fists across their hearts. (Australia's Peter Norman, the silver medallist, gave mute support, wearing an American civil rights badge). 'I was tossed up as the patriotic guy', Foreman told me. 'A lot of people bugged me about it. I got a chip on my shoulder from the criticism but it was the happiest day of my life.'

Foreman is opposed to sport being a vehicle of political protest and, to him, the futility of the Black Power protest was demonstrated only four years later. 'How successful were Smith and Carlos in the end?' he asked rhetorically, his seeming innocuousness sheathing an arrow that hits its mark. 'What happened? Munich and all the bloodshed! Let athletes play games undisturbed by political demonstrations. Sure, there are social problems to be fixed but not through protests.'

It's a complex debate. If you accept George Santayana's maxim—that those who fail to remember the past are condemned to repeat it—you could argue that the organisers of the 1970 Games, where athletes were housed in a village not that distant from the World War II Dachau concentration camp, recalled their past all too well, thereby inviting a horror of a different sort. Furthermore, when terrorists attacked the Sri Lankan cricket team in Pakistan, the world took notice. Bombings and shootings happen almost daily in Pakistan but, when sport becomes involved, the story dominates global news. Terrorists use sport as a stage to publicise their grievances, but do athletes really care?

The United Arab Emirates decision to deny a visa to an Israeli tennis player, Shahar Pe'er, to prevent her competing in the 2009 Dubai Open, did not raise any reaction on the social conscience meter. One of the world's leading female players, Venus Williams, an African-American raised in the slums of Compton, California, said no player would boycott the tournament because, 'There are too many other people involved. Sponsors are important to us.' Pe'er also sought to distance herself from the debate, saying diplomatically she expected the Women's Tennis Association would act to protect her from future injustices. Insofar as the WTA consists of her fellow professionals, she couldn't expect much support. She was also naive when she said, 'There should be no place for politics or discrimination in professional tennis or any other sport'. Sport could not exist without politics.

Pe'er was allowed to play in 2010 Dubai Open on the condition she stayed away from other players' hotels and travelled to the tennis centre from her hotel under tight security. She reached the semifinal, playing Venus Williams on the middle of three courts, with fans confined to the far side of one of the adjacent courts and TV cameras stationed on the far side of the other adjacent court. Pe'er lost in straight sets and declinded to enter the political debate, saying she had achieved 'a lot professional for myself and also mentally, for my inside'.

The reality is that professional athletes of all persuasions are too self-absorbed to care much for social causes. Evidence of the self-centred view of footballers is the toothlessness of players' unions, unless financed by, say, the AFL. And this resourcing is usually on the understanding that the Indians won't take legal action against the chiefs to challenge an essential regulator of competition, such as the salary cap or the draft.

When Ali stood at the vortex of history and announced he had become a Muslim and refused induction into the US Army, it became a rallying cry for millions. There has been no-one to rival him since. Ask today's athletes about their stance and they'll explain how they position themself under a high ball, or shape up to the bowler at the crease. Stuart MacGill, who refused to tour Zimbabwe with the Australian cricket team in 2002, may well be the last cricketer to act on his social conscience.

SIX

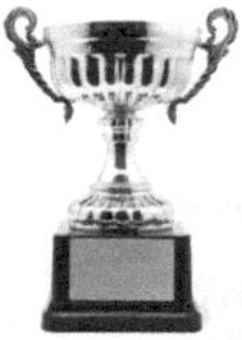

SLEAZIER

John Landy, the gentle middle-distance runner, was watching a track-and-field meeting at Olympic Park, Melbourne, when a mutual friend mentioned that the 40th anniversary of the fabled 1956 Australian mile championship at the same venue had passed without mention in the media. This was the race where Landy stopped to help the fallen Ron Clarke to his feet and then returned to the track, caught his opponents and won. Twenty-two thousand people, a record for the small ground, witnessed Landy's generosity of spirit. By stopping, he lost 60 metres on his opponents and still won by nine. His time was four minutes 4.2 seconds. Reporters in the press box, usually consumed with deadline dread, stood and clapped.

When the friend—Melbourne *Herald Sun* journalist, Ron Reed—told Landy the anniversary of the 11 March 1956 event had gone unheralded, Landy turned to us with a mixture of relief and scorn on his face and said, 'Thank Christ'. Landy has always claimed the media has made too much of it. His gesture merely meant he missed running the first sub-four-minute mile on his hometown track. A loss would not have meant missing his hometown Olympics, where qualification is over 1500 metres. Yet decades later, a statue has been erected within the shadows of the MCG honouring the occasion.

Perhaps Landy, a self-effacing former Governor of Victoria whose hobby is collecting butterflies, thinks we make too much of sport. After all, organised sport is the increasing perfection of the unnecessary—its purpose is to do something which doesn't need doing better than someone else has done it. Landy spent his early adulthood in pursuit of perfecting the unnecessary: he was the second person to break the four-minute mile, eclipsing Englishman Roger Bannister's time set six weeks earlier.

Sport, unlike art and music, is one of the rare fields of human achievement where it's possible to measure improvement. We have become destroyers of distance and thieves of time: running faster, leaping higher, throwing further, lifting heavier weights and swimming quicker . . . all quantifiable measures. Perhaps Landy believes that by placing sport on a pedestal, we've made too much of it.

In the half century since his heyday, there has been an explosion in the importance we attach to all major sports to the point where teams have become civic metaphors and ordinary athletes elevated to spokesmen for social causes. The results of individual games have become a point of national importance. Indeed, El Salvador and Honduras went to war in 1969 over a soccer game. And wasn't it Australian Prime Minister Bob Hawke who told the nation after we won the America's Cup yacht race in 1983, 'Any boss who sacks a worker for not turning up today is a bum'?

Landy's race against Bannister at the 1954 Vancouver Commonwealth Games was billed as the 'Mile of the Century' and yet there was still another 46 years of the century to run. Perhaps he has seen enough hyperbole. Or is Landy's dismissive view of history linked to a very human quality: is he miffed at forever being reminded of the Clarke race and his record of coming second to Bannister—he took the silver medal in Vancouver—rather than his other great achievements? Or could it be Landy doesn't go along with the nineteenth century ideal, perpetuated by the statue, that sport is central to the development of character? After all, that belief was pushed by the English nobles who were the only ones with the time to pursue sport, most of which was spent on horseback chasing foxes with the help of dogs. ('The unspeakable in full pursuit of the uneatable', as Oscar Wilde put it.)

My view is that Landy recognises the essential hypocrisy of our adulation at his act of stopping to help Clarke. Would we have celebrated Landy if he had lost? Are we honouring sportsmanship when we are really honouring winning? At least the statue of Landy and Clarke celebrates something that actually happened, as opposed to what we assumed took place. Rugby league's premiership trophy—depicting the two mud-caked 1963 Sydney first-grade grand-final captains, St George's Norm Provan and Western Suburbs' Arthur Summons—allegedly honours sportsmanship. It's an image of two rivals, arms linked at the end of a tough battle—one tall and the other short—representing a game that caters for all shapes and sizes. Their jerseys are so indistinguishable in the mud that they could be team mates walking off together, rather than combatants simultaneously consoling and congratulating. The mud also symbolises the importance of sport and its grand finals—the game must go on, even if the weather is about the only variable we can't control these days. Well, other than the bounce of the ball . . . and some stars, such as the retired rugby league hero, Andrew Johns, could even control that.

Much of this symbolism of the trophy is true, except what was being said by the captains at the time. Summons told the media at rugby league's 100-year anniversary party: 'He wanted to swap jumpers and I told him to get stuffed and that St George not only beat us but the referee was paid to do a job on us.' Not a Western Suburbs reunion goes by without some mention of the referee on that 1963 sky-saturated Saturday afternoon, Darcy Lawler. Lawler was then the boss of South Sydney Juniors, one of the first of the big poker-machine palaces and also the haunt of Sydney's criminal milieu. Wests players insist St George winger, Johnny King, was tackled but allowed to rise to his feet without playing the ball and run to the tryline and score.

Grainy vision of the match does show the Wests players stopping, as if they'd heard Lawler tell King to play the ball. It was the Magpies third successive grand final loss to the Dragons and would have interrupted St George's eleven successive premierships, a run which ended in 1967. Because I attend reunions of both clubs, I hear both sides. The Wests players are still bitter, while it's rarely mentioned at Kogarah, except to say, 'Look at the scoreboard.'

The photo from which the trophy was sculptured and the piece itself also have unhappy histories. Fairfax photographer, John O'Gready, never believed he was given sufficient credit, or any financial reward for his outstanding picture. A *Sun-Herald* editor actually discarded the photo for the Sunday edition of the paper and it was first used in the Monday *Sydney Morning Herald*.

Rothmans, the tobacco company that sponsored rugby league at the time, commissioned a sculptor, Alan Ingham, to create a piece based on the photo and called it the Winfield Cup, after the name of a brand of cigarettes formed from the two words 'win' and 'field'. Ingham completed the Winfield Cup over six months in 1982 in his Newport studio. He told me early in 1993, when he was 72 and suffering from advanced prostate cancer, 'I have felt guilty about the Winfield Cup as the years go by. I am not proud of it as a piece of work. Firstly, it is based on a photograph and, secondly, the public links the trophy with smoking. I'm anti-smoking and I don't want to have anything more to do with it. I sold Rothmans the copyright and gave them the originals and the mould and I've wiped my hands clean of it. I only asked for $1500. My need was to get rid of it. My sympathy is with the journalists who refer to the premiership trophy as the Giltinan Shield, rather than the Winfield Cup.'

The Giltinan Shield, a separate trophy, was named after J.J. Giltinan, the founder of rugby league in Australia—for a time, the NSWRL premiership winner received both trophies. The Giltinan Shield is now awarded to the minor premier and the major premier receives the Provan–Summons trophy, although it is called a cup and named after Telstra, or whoever holds the naming rights to the NRL.

Ingham may have had another motivation in preferring the name Giltinan. His only hope of staying alive at the time lay in the hands of a medical researcher at Sydney's Prince of Wales Hospital, Professor Pam Russell, who headed a team committed to finding out why one in nineteen Australian males suffered from prostate cancer. Professor Russell told me, 'I'm a Giltinan. My grandfather was a Catholic from Sydney and married a Methodist from Tasmania and they got cut off from both families. My grandfather was the brother of the founder of rugby league.' So, by a curious coincidence, the life of a man who sculptured a trophy he loathed rested in the hands of a descendant of the man whose memory was being marginalised by the trophy. Ingham told me he would like to see a Mark II version of the Giltinan Shield. He said that if Professor Russell could discover a technique that protected all Australian men from the disease killing him, it would be the best Giltinan Shield imaginable.

Shortly after meeting Ingham, I attended a Fairfax boardroom lunch with the top executives of the rugby league administration and passed on Professor Russell's comments about the abysmal lack of money for medical research in Australia. She lamented that the NSW Cancer Council had a bias towards female cancer, such as pap smears and mammography campaigns and little research was being carried out on prostate cancer, principally because the disease is a concomitant of old age and many doctors rationalise that men have to die some time. I argued that if rugby league is a game principally played by men and prostate cancer kills only men, the NSWRL should nominate Professor Russell's research as its principal charity. The idea was firmly rejected by the league chiefs, who claimed it would invite a flood of requests from other charities.

So the years rolled by and rugby league didn't have an official medical charity until it joined the NSW Cancer Council's 'bias' and embraced research into breast cancer. In the intervening years, the wives of two leading players had died from breast cancer and the NRL was also keen to demonstrate its feminine side, particularly when it came under fire following reports of sexual assault and sleaze. To celebrate Women in League week 2009, Penrith became the 'Pink Panthers' for a match against Manly, dressing in pink from their boots to the tips of their pink beards.

The idealisation of sport represented in these two pieces of statuary could tempt us into the oft-expressed view sport is like life. But sport is not like life, irrespective of what your mini league or Minkey hockey coach told you. Games are wonderfully unlike life: they have set beginnings and ends, precise rules, a fixed number of balls per over or tackles per set, prescribed boundaries and points, referees and umpires, grades of penalties and—at the final whistle-siren or signal from an official—losers and winners. One of sports essential charms is it produces black and white results in a world dappled in grey.

One sport that tries to convince us that it is like life is golf. Thomas Friedman wrote in the *New York Times*, 'Baseball, basketball and football are played on flat surfaces designed to give true bounces. [Friedman's "football" must refer to the round-ball game of soccer.] Golf is played on an uneven terrain designed to surprise. Good and bad bounces are built into the essence of the game. And the reason golf is so much like life is that the game—like life—is all about how you react to those good and bad bounces. Do you blame your caddy? Do you cheat? Do you throw your clubs? Or do you accept it with dignity and grace and move on, as Tom Watson always has. Hence the saying: Play one round of golf with someone and you will learn everything you need to know about his character.'

The story golfers cite is Bobby Jones penalising himself a stroke during the 1925 US Open. He accidentally nudged his golf ball less than an inch when addressing it deep in the rough. He called the marshals over and announced he had hit the ball. He missed by one stroke on winning the tournament outright and then lost a playoff. When praised for his sportsmanship, Jones said, 'You may as well praise me for not robbing a bank.'

Jones had the certainty of the rule book. We don't have that certainty in life, either with the health of our families, or in the security of our jobs, or in the course of our economy and its interest and employment rates. We can continue for years living a mundane, equivocal existence but the games of athletes are yes and no. In fact, the only time sportspeople complain about the conduct of their games is when they lack certainty, that is, when 'the 50:50 calls', as they term them—where the referee can rule in favour of either side—go against them. The rest of us look for certainty in our lives because with it comes confidence, contentment and peace. It follows that winners in games appear to have what we seek most. The sport-is-like-life argument seduces us into believing athletes make great role models.

So how must the 'golf-is-like-Tiger' people have felt when the world's best golfer/role model/first sport billionaire was exposed for his sleazy secret life? His nickname changed to 'Tom Cat', then a 'Cheetah' chasing Cougars. Woods took the largest ratings plunge in Gallup Poll history. He had a 33 per cent 'favourable' rating in the days following the revelation he was a serial adulterer, compared to the 85 per cent mark in 2005 when the question was last posed. His fall mirrored that of ex-US President George W. Bush.

Writers recalled the quote of Tiger's late father, Earl, who famously said his purpose in raising Tiger was 'not to raise a golfer. I want to raise a good person.' Others resurrected a letter Tiger wrote to young golfers in 'Tiger's Action Plan', a program of the Tiger Woods Foundation: 'If you are open to it, there is so much that will make you a great friend, a great team mate, a great son or daughter, a great brother or sister, a great student and, most important, a great person.' Perhaps these words were written by Tiger's management team but if athletes allow minders to control and manipulate their image, they are complicit when the hypocrisy is revealed.

The Woods affair sent a chilling message to all elite sportspeople and those who sponsor them, such as Gillette, which turned Tiger into a corporate totem and then toppled him. Exposure is a double-edged sword, as fine a blade as any manufactured by Mr Gillette. The stunning advertising campaigns deliver millions of dollars to the athlete but he becomes vulnerable to temptation and sex traps and a public who wants to know what is behind that heavenly smile and steely eyes.

The problem is that footballers, cricket players, basketballers and now golfers have achieved their certainty in a world different to ours. Because someone is nearly two metres tall and can run fast, jump high in the lineout or over the bar, dunk a ball or knock a six over the stadium clock, we believe he or she is someone to be revered and emulated. Someone whose words are to be devoured and whose clothes should be copied. Yet none of their physical skills have much value away from the playing venue.

Sportspeople have attained their self-confidence in a sure, structured world that has little to do with the real world. But our own lives on the assembly line or the farm or in the office or home duties are often characterised by a tedium that is broken only by the thrill and colour of the weekend. Yet we demand our athletic heroes be our role models.

When the Crawford Report into future federal government funding of sport was released late in 2009, recommending a re-direction of money away from Olympic sports, AOC chairman John Coates countered by saying Olympic heroes inspire a nation. This argument only holds if you accept athletes are role models. It also explains why the AOC has demanded a higher level of behaviour from Olympic athletes than could reasonably be expected of citizens the same age. My strong view is that if you wear an

Australian blazer, or a St George rugby league jumper, receive a grant courtesy of the taxpayer, or spruik for Weeties, you better behave as nicely as a young boy eating his breakfast cereal. Even fifteen-year-old schooboys understand this.

When Shane Warne was enjoying a rich sponsorship from a manufacturer of nicotine patches, an adolescent with a camera in New Zealand photographed him smoking. On an earlier tour of the West Indies, Warne brazenly smoked cigarettes and cigars in front of the cricket writers; when he got nearer to home and under closer media and particularly TV scrutiny, his double standards were more likely to be exposed. When the young photographer snapped Warne with a cigarette in Wellington, the world's greatest-ever bowler remonstrated with the lad, drawing further attention to his lucrative deceit. Warne couldn't be accused of hypocrisy when he sleazily pursued sexy women by mobile phone, but there's little doubt he was better equipped to roll models than be one.

While most elite sportsmen hate the role-model argument, the cricketers and footballers who do welcome the responsibility tend to represent minorities. The NRL Bulldogs' Hazem El Masri, Australian rugby league's record points scorer, has also received the code's annual award for community work. When he was photographed receiving the NRL's Women in League's 'Favourite Son' award, accompanied by his wife who was wearing a hijab, it sent a 'Not all Muslims are terrorists' message to the rednecks. Similarly, the community work of Aboriginal AFL stars, while genuine, also has the effect of saying, 'We are a world away from petrol sniffers.'

Swimmer Ian Thorpe recognised the hypocrisy of athletes being used to promote social causes when he plunged headfirst into Australia's failure to address the problems of our indigenous communities. Speaking at a Beyond Sport Summit in London in July 2009, Thorpe commented on a realisation that came to him after becoming, at fifteen, the youngest-ever male world swimming champion. He told the audience, 'I realised my value to organisations trying to bring positive change lent enormous weight to these causes. I must say, though, this should be an outrage, because as an athlete I am not qualified to comment on health or education as the health professionals and educators who daily tackle the big issues. In fact it is a bit disappointing that a teenager's opinion garnered more attention than those who had been working on their chosen causes before I was even born.'

In the main, men in male professional team sports resent the higher standards society and sports officials demand of their behaviour. They claim they were never trained to be role models. Rugby league legend and later NRL board member, Gorden Tallis, once asked me, 'Where is it in the school curriculum that you learn to be a role model?' They recognise the hypocrisy of sport bosses asking them to assist in the promotion of alcohol, gambling and fast food, while at the same time demanding they be role models.

When a rugby league footballer is photographed via a mobile phone as he urinates behind the back wall of a pub, and then is fined $10,000 by his club because a newspaper that half-owns the NRL puts it on page three in order to increase sales, he is entiled to raise at least one eyebrow. He loathes being told the justification for this punishment—twenty times greater than what a normal citizen would receive—is because he is a role model. He even understands the intrinsic conflict of an organisation using the photograph to sell newspapers, while aware it is diminishing the value of the asset it half-owns and is obliged—via a contract—to eventually sell. I suspect the role-model argument has turned footballers into blame takers. We live in an age where fewer people are taking responsibility for their own actions. So, when a teenage footballer pisses behind a pub, his parents excuse his behaviour, saying, 'what would you expect when NRL heroes do it!'

Some sports, such as swimming, embrace the role-model argument and support zero tolerance of drugs and alcohol bans. Perhaps it's no coincidence swimming has enjoyed lucrative sponsorships from Australian companies with a 'motherhood' image. The sport's banning of Nick D'Arcy from the Beijing Olympics—for punching a retired swimmer and breaking his jaw—could be seen to be protecting that wholesome image. Indeed, perhaps the greatest athlete–role model in the history of Australian sport is swimmer, Susie O'Neill—who else would stand down as a member of the International Olympic Committee, declining all its privileges, because the travel took them away from their partner and children?

Footballers point to those in more pastoral roles in society, such as politicians and clergymen, who offend and receive less punishment. They argue politicians get pissed, take bribes, drive while drunk, strangle each other in the party room and are caught out in the bedroom, yet their punishments aren't as severe. Insofar as the pollies are elected as the representative of hundreds of thousands of people, aren't they role models, too?

When an amateur Aussie Rules team in Melbourne, from the Prahran club, was outed by a Melbourne newspaper in 2009 for hiring a stripper to perform before a game, the politicians went beserk. Premier Brumby raged about this immoral behaviour, while Prime Minister Rudd stood beside him, nodding in harmony at the diatribe. This was the same Rudd who once attended a strip club in New York in company with an Australian-born editor of a Gotham City tabloid and was too drunk to recall the stage show. The politicians couldn't sensibly use the role-model argument against the Prahran fourths, because they were hardly an elite team. However, this incident came shortly after a *Four Corners* report on group sex that had tectonic impact and the politicians were suddenly keen to be heard on the topic of the degradation of women.

The ABC-TV report had focused on an episode which occurred seven years earlier in Christchurch during a short pre-season tour by the NRL's Cronulla Sharks. Matthew Johns, by then a broken-down 31-year-old five eighth, had been party to a gang bang, or 'bun' as they are known in rugby league, with a nineteen-year-old kitchen hand. Five days after this incident, the girl had complained to local NZ police and they had flown to Sydney and interviewed over 40 players and staff, before deciding no charges would be laid. The media had known at the time that Johns was one of the players involved, but they were also aware he had told his wife. Furthermore, the police would not reveal the girl's name and newspaper budgets don't allow reporters to jump on planes to Christchurch, so the episode went largely unreported.

When this episode was re-visited by *Four Corners*, Johns was at the top of the TV tree as a host of the prime-time *Footy Show*. He was encouraged by both the show's producer and his own manager to take a pre-emptive strike against the ABC by admitting to the incident on the show, four days before the *Four Corners* report went to air. Channel Nine did not count on the New Zealand woman's testimony. It was harrowing; she wanted to kill the men involved. It was portrayed as the ultimate degradation of women.

It eclipsed standard sleaze. It conjured up images of the sickening, humiliating treatment of Iraqi prisoners by soldiers for the Coalition of the Willing. Johns' position on TV and as an assistant coach became untenable and he resigned.

The *Four Corners* report explored the issue of group sex as a bonding exercise and the ABC reporter grilled me on this during a 90-minute interview that was later edited down. It's true that group sex is sometimes a bonding phenomenon but it's hard to say this on TV without creating an impression you endorse it, particularly if you are an ex-coach and the program is edited. The notion of players standing around half-naked, drinking beer, waiting their turn with a girl behind the closed door of the bedroom excites the essayists on the opinion pages of the broadsheets who invariably link this with homoerotic tendencies. They argue players shower together, tape each other's ankles, walk around nude in the dressing room, so they conclude group sex with a woman is a substitute for what they'd like to do with a man. They downplay the motives of the Cougars, as predatory women are called, or of the American beauty who farewelled a group of Sydney footballers on an end-of-season trip to Hawaii in the early 1980s with, 'I can't wait to get back to the States and tell my friends I was fucked by a football team.'

It's also important to point out the vast majority of footballers elect to have nothing to do with group sex, but they do seek each other out away from the football field. They genuinely enjoy each other's company and anything which unites them—such as, a night at the movies, paintball, a fishing trip, a day at the races—they embrace. Okay, such relatively innocent outings are a far cry from group sex, but sexual satisfaction isn't the aim of this sleazy exercise, during which the guys laugh at the sexually incompetent—the ones who are flaccid or, more particularly, the ones rejected by the girl because they are ugly, or awarded a mark of one out of ten by her for their lack of sexual prowess. The sex isn't equalizing; rather it's the intimacy within the tribe, being 'one of the boys' which is the bonding mechanism. Furthermore, when the girl is giving them marks for degree of difficulty, like dives being scored off the high-board, she is the one with the power in the room.

But the Christchurch case, and another involving the Bulldogs in Coffs Harbour in 2004, highlighted the more usual phenomenon—when men have the power and the woman has none. The Christchurch girl went willingly to the hotel room with two players, but not with the additional half dozen or so who later joined them. The Coffs Harbour girl became hysterical when the players abandoned her on the eve of returning to Sydney and one of them had earlier called her a 'slut'. The way the Coffs Harbour girl was treated—which was exposed by the media the day after it happened—angered many ex-players, some of whom may have participated in group sex in the past but had done so according to whatever rules were laid down by the woman involved.

The *Four Corners* program was privately criticised in the league community for bias and quotations taken out of context but the revelations were so horrendous that the code's leaders could say little in response. The wider media did buy into the debate, wondering why the Christchurch woman suddenly allowed herself to be interviewed while many of her former workmates at the hotel were not questioned by the ABC. 'We need never fear an objective appraisal of our heroes', Thomas Reeves wrote in *A Question of Character*, an analysis of American President John

F. Kennedy and the lore that surrounds him. 'Truth is ultimately more enlightening and satisfying than myth.' True, but no-one ever exposed JFK for his sexual dalliances during his presidency, despite an entire press corps knowing about it.

In the firestorm of publicity after the *Four Corners* program, John Elliott mentioned during a forum at a football lunch in Tasmania that five women had been paid $5000 each as hush money for rapes committed in 1999 during his presidency of AFL club Carlton. The Melbourne media joined the AFL in reviling Elliott, labelling him a dinosaur. A one-time prime ministerial aspirant and Liberal Party president, he was accussed of what former Attorney-General Gareth Evans calls 'Relevance Deprivation Syndrome.' Despite one of the rape victims providing Melbourne radio stations and newspapers with her own personal account of these events, only the ABC's *7.30 Report* gave any space/time to her story.

Elliott was ridiculed but no-one said it wasn't true. The same year, he did not receive the two grand final tickets the AFL routinely send to life members. Carlton's then president, Stephen Kernahan, was forced to do a deal with his old friend, where Elliott had to stay away from the club. Kernahan was quoted saying, 'While John harbours such opinions, he will not be welcome at the club and he will not be permitted to attend any official Carlton Football Club functions.' To merge two very appropriate clichés: Elliott was sent to Coventry in a classic case of shooting the messenger.

Ironically, the *Four Corners* program that exposed the rugby league cases of sexual assault was entitled 'Code of Silence.' But it did not have time to investigate the AFL, which did its best to bury the 1999 case. There is irony in the reason for the short turnaround time *Four Corners* had in getting the program to air.

Initially, it was interested in finding a subject of interest in the northern states, while the southern states could be expected to be watching commercial TV's first Monday night game of the 2009 AFL season. So *Four Corners* only had time to focus on one code of football while the AFL states were watching the best of another. As it transpired, *Four Corners* had time to fly to Tokyo and interview the woman at the centre of the Christchurch affair. It also generated sufficient material to consider running 'Code of Silence' Part 1 and 2 on consecutive Monday nights.

The program won the 2009 Walkely Award for sports journalism. Johns' colleague at Channel Nine, Tracy Grimshaw, also won, a Walkely for best TV interview. It was a harrowing interrogation in which Johns, under contract to the network and in the prescence of his wife Trish, relived the sleazy incident. He resigned from Nine shortly afterwards and later sacked his manager. It was a classic case of the media eating one of its own but the overwhelming view was that if this was necessary to rid the game of sleaze, Johns was a fair sacrifice. Johns subsequently returned to TV a year later on a rival network. The rugby league community willed *The Matty Johns Show* to be a success but the early prime-time ratings indicated many women had not forgiven him.

Sportspeople bond with each other in ways the rest of society can never understand. In the main, they like each other—more than say, schoolteachers or journalists or clergymen enjoy each other's company. Perhaps it is the shared agony of knowing how much a tackle hurt, or that a referee's ruling was unjust, or a selector's decision unfair, or that the bounce of a ball was just plain unlucky. They know games can be won by a ball rebounding off the fresh coat of paint on a crossbar.

While it's true 'winners are grinners and the losers can please themselves', players empathise with opponents who have lost a game through bad luck. One of the most memorable instances of this is the occasion English bowler Andrew Flintoff consoled Australian batsman Brett Lee at the end of the 2005 Edgbaston Test, when Australia lost by two runs. Lee had batted magnificently and almost pulled it off—or 'got out of jail', or 'burgled it', as is sometimes said. It was the loss that set up England's Test series win; but Flintoff had compassion for Lee, left alone at the crease when his batting partner was given out. 'At the end of the day, we're only cattle', footballers often say, meaning they have more in common with the enemy than with their own administration which is willing to sell them for a transfer fee, or in order to relieve salary cap pressure.

It follows that a footballer can swap clubs and immediately be welcomed by those whom he sledged and savaged the previous season. Rugby league's inaugural State of Origin game in 1980 achieved instant credibility when Sydney clubmates belted each other in the opening minutes, demonstrating the fluidity and pragmatism of sporting friendships. That 1980 night and succeeding years, the 'state against state, mate against mate' mantra meant something, unlike the end-of-season all-star games in American sports, in which their core promise of The Best Versus The Best is betrayed. The US public perceives these games, such as the NFL's 'Pro Bowl', for what they are—players being rewarded for a season's work by being chosen for a showcase game which does little more than deliver some incentive clauses in a contract.

Rugby union's Barbarian games, in which an international all-star cast is gathered to play a national team, are highly competitive. The original Barbarians Club dates back to the 1880s and involved men from different British clubs going away on an Easter tour. However, the classic Barbarian fixtures occur at the end of tours of the British Isles by any national team from Australia, New Zealand and South Africa. These games assume even greater importance if the touring team has been undefeated, as occurred in January 1961, at the end of the Springboks' five month tour of the United Kingdom.

The 1960–61 South African team was one of the most unpopular touring teams in the history of the sport, playing a dour, win-at-all-costs style. The Barbarian selectors responded by choosing a team with the sole object of beating the undefeated Springboks at their own game. They assembled a disparate collection of men of all nationalities—except South African—all equally at home with a take-no-prisoners style. The Barbarians won, ruining the Springboks' perfect record. However, the first of these end-of-tour Barbarians games was conceived in a different fashion.

The 1947–48 Wallabies were keen to return to Australia from Great Britain via the United States and Canada, playing games on the way, but they had run out of money. The Barbarians Club agreed to stage a match and give the Wallabies a slice of the gate in order for them to visit North America. From that first game, played in the best spirit of the then amateur code, came a tradition of hard-fought contests. Perhaps there was a social contract drawn up from that first game, as a consciousness among men who were to become leaders in business, medicine and the law: 'If you are good enough to pay to watch us play a game put on to benefit us, we'll put on a good show.'

Compare this to the Barbarians match played in Sydney in 2009, the first time a 'Bar-Bar' match, as they are called, was played in Australia. Former rugby league star Sonny Bill Williams, then signed with a French rugby union club, was selected in the Barbarians team to play the Wallabies, with the match staged a few days after league's annual first State of Origin match. The Australian Rugby Union effectively sent a message to league: 'Look at who we have raining on your parade.' It was a cynical exercise from a less-than-committed Barbarians team, as the Wallabies' one-sided victory demonstrated.

Other sports, such as tennis and cricket, have demonstrated that players can be geographically disparate, and yet come together a few days before an event and quickly gel. Australia's Lleyton Hewitt is a highly motivated individual but he refuses to miss a Davis Cup tie. The welcomed opportunity to be a member of an Australian tennis team at a Grand Slam tournament, even if playing against each other in the final, dates back to post-World War II Wimbledon. Our players, many of them parsimonious, would stay at a cheap London pub, buy beer from the off licence, cool it in the bathtub and drink together after matches. This tradition began with Frank Sedgman who passed the torch—or was it a bottle of pilsener?—to Lew Hoad . . . to Rod Laver . . . to John Newcombe, who tried to instill this camaraderie in modern Davis Cup teams but was undermined by the rise of the tennis entourage. These tennis hangers-on, following the star, make up a tail longer than Halley's Comet. They have given the circuit the look of a travelling rock tour. Pat Cash won a Davis Cup for Australia; but he also won Wimbledon with a brain and body health squad identified by their checkered headbands, an idea inspired by his personal psychologist.

Just as tennis players will attempt to destroy their opponents in singles matches and then bond with their former opponents in Davis Cup teams, IPL players who once reviled each other in Test matches, now play on the same Indian teams. But this is not a new phenomenon in cricket. In 1970, when the South African team's tour of England was cancelled because of the evil apartheid policy of its government, the authorities replaced it with a series of matches between England and a multiracial Rest of the World team, led by West Indian Gary Sobers. Sobers' selection reinforced the message that apartheid was anathema to the rest of the cricket world. The Rest of the World team also included Indian and Pakistani players, but war broke out between their nations during the series. This allowed sport to send yet a further message—almost a press release to the world—which said, if we can play together, our countries should be able to get along.

Similarly, a match was staged at the MCG in January 2005 in the wake of the tsunami that swept through the Pacific and South Asia. Muralitharan, the only Tamil in the Sri Lankan team, agreed to return to Australia for the first time since he had been no-balled in the country and the game was a great success. However, the ICC Super Series of 2005, in which Australia played a Rest of the World team in three One Day Internationals and a Test nine months later, did not capture the interests of anyone. The Champion Team versus the Team of Champions concept, played without any worthy social cause, was perceived to be a phoney and commercially driven.

Yet cricket has probably produced the best example ever of former enemies embracing. English fast bowler Harold Larwood, the man ordered to dispatch bouncers at Bradman, later migrated to Sydney with his family. During England's 1932–33 Bodyline tour of Australia, Larwood took 33 wickets at an average of nineteen runs and England regained the Ashes 4–1. Larwood, who had been ordered to bowl short at the batsman's body by his captain, Douglas

Jardine, was later asked to sign a letter of apology for employing such unsporting tactics. He refused and never played another Test. He retired to run a sweet shop in Blackpool but an old adversary from Australia, Jack Fingleton, encouraged him to join the tide of migrants coming to Australia post World War II. Larwood lived in Sydney for 45 years until his death at age 90, warmly embraced by the nation which once wanted to lynch him.

The way sport bonds athletes, particularly victorious teams, was keenly evident to me when I flew to Adelaide in late 1987 with members of the Australian cricket team that had toured England in 1948. I was attending the launch of the *Bradman Albums*. Bradman, after considerable scrutiny of the pages written, had reluctantly agreed that his career be memorialised in a series of books launched almost 40 years after the team's unbeaten tour. My sports editor thought it was a great idea for the recently retired St George rugby league coach to accompany the cricketers to Adelaide and perhaps snare an interview with Bradman, who had played grade cricket for St George when he moved from Bowral to Sydney early in his career. I had also corresponded with Bradman in my capacity as a board member of the ASC, encouraging him to publicly back Aussie Sports, a program of modified sport for primary school children. I subsequently framed his letters which show his pedantry, chiding me for not dating one 'epistle' as he called it and altering the punctuation in his message of support for the project.

My problem with the Adelaide trip was our Ansett free flight left at 7 am and we subsequently spent all day at the bar and the new Adelaide casino. Little Lindsay Hassett, the vice-captain of that team and later Australian captain, looking like a beaming ET (from the popular movie of five years earlier), was the treasurer of the afternoon drinking session.

The ex-players related with each other as if 1948 was yesterday and exchanged yarns, many of them about Bradman, whom they knew they would not see until the dinner that evening, even though Adelaide was his home town. Everyone came down with a bad case of nostalgia, with stories focusing on biased umpires, grog and girls. 'Why did you tell that German nurse I was married when I wasn't?' one asked. By 7 pm, they all wore the wobbly boot.

Dressing for the dinner represented a problem for spin bowler Doug Ring, who in the absence of 'the missus' needed Ernie Toshack to tie his black tie. Ring suffered a heart attack during the dinner and his mates made bumbling attempts to revive him with mouth-to-mouth resuscitation and cardiac massage. 'He was gone', Ray Lindwall told me as Ring lay on a stretcher waiting for the ambulance. Lindwall's fellow fast bowler, Keith Miller, was more circumspect, leaning down every ten minutes or so, beer glass in hand, saying to his pale team mate, 'All right, Dougie?' Bill Johnstone accompanied Ring to hospital, where he recovered. Meanwhile, Toshack responded to anyone's observation that Ring 'looked crook', with the statement, 'He should be bloody crook, too. He's been on the grog with me all afternoon.'

Sir Donald, positioned only one table away, was the only member of the 1948 team to remain seated during Ring's collapse. Sitting hawk-like, wizened, sipping cold water and signing autographs, Bradman maintained his distance from a team he described as 'the greatest cricket team to have ever played'. A colour portrait of the Don was auctioned to raise money for charity. It showed a classic Bradman cover drive; but he was critical of the positioning of his hands, claiming they should have been a quarter of an inch closer to the bat. When it went for $13,000, an inebriated guest yelled out to the successful bidder, 'You've paid $13,000 and he got out with that shot.' Bradman quietly muttered, 'No, I did not.'

It seemed as if he remembered every one of his 6996 runs in 52 Tests. He said of his 254 at Lords in 1930, 'It was my best innings. Apart from one or two exceptions, every ball went where I expected it to go. It was the nearest to technical perfection.' But the single-minded, disciplined qualities that made Bradman great did not endear him to his team mates. He was a generation older than most of the 1948 team; perhaps he was the Richard III of cricket—the more you knew him, the less you liked him. He must have been great because he endured, despite choosing to distance himself from the team.

When the 1930s team returned from his record-breaking tour of England, Bradman's employer, sports supplier Mick Simmons, flew him from Perth, where the ship first docked, to Sydney ahead of the rest of the touring party. Bradman was treated as a hero on his arrival in Sydney, but he disappointed his team mates who claimed no-one wanted to know them when they eventually arrived fourteen days later. He also used a tour of America and Canada during the winter of 1932 as his honeymoon. In his defence, it should be remembered he told the Australian Cricket Board he didn't want to tour—it not being fair on his wife—but the board persisted because he was the star. After laying down a number of conditions, he boarded the ship with his wife and enjoyed the privileges of first class. However, the rest of the team made no money from the tour and to avoid the embarrassment of not being able to tip porters, they took to sneaking down the gangway when it was unattended.

Lindwall summed up the story of Bradman and his team the day following the launch of the albums. 'They presented Bradman with ten books,' he said. 'We got none. But still . . . the books are all about him.'

Today's players derive pleasure within the cocoon of each other's company, but the danger inherent in this is they thus remove themselves from contact with society's mores. Many are not exposed to the socialising influence of females—they move straight from a schoolboy football factory to the professional team where they are insulated from the mothers, wives, sisters, daughters, aunts and even grandmothers who once flocked to the clubhouse after games. When they do receive lectures on treating women, or on drugs, or post-career education, some look out the window.

Footballers are not social scientists, or cultural historians. Quite the contrary. The truth is we want them to do the right thing because they inherently know it is the right thing, not because society demands it. Yet their upbringing and schooling often excludes education on what is the right thing. Part of the problem is that the very best of them have tunnel vision. They create an insular fortress in which all considerations beyond the game itself are feared to carry the contamination of what coaches and even the media call 'distractions'. Focus is their god. After all, their tasks on the field are simple and only require reflection when they make an error. Indeed, second-guessing oneself is the athlete's mortal enemy.

Great athletes are a lot like children—naive, self-centred and highly competitive. They rise to representative teams and drop to reserve grade on the outcome of simple events: a ball off the edge of the bat, a lucky bounce, a missed tackle. It's the real world that really worries them. Star athletes fall the hardest when the simplicity of their calling collides with the complexity of the adult world, when they lose out to deceitful investors, devious journalists, breathalysers, sex traps and gambling.

They must also be on the lookout for the 'trapperazzi'—the drunk who throws a punch so his mate can capture the retaliatory blow on his mobile phone camera, or the female accomplice who snaps him fondling her friend. Footballers admit to photographing casual sex on their own phones as evidence it was consensual in the event of a later cry of rape. This shrewd tactic would seem to refute the view, especially amongst social elitists who follow cricket and rugby union, that rugby league and AFL are more prone to social accidents because their practitioners are of lower intelligence. That is more wishful thinking than reality.

It is worth remembering cricketers and rugby union players usually don't cement a place in elite squads—such as Test teams, or even franchises such as the Brumbies, Reds, Waratahs and Western Force—until they are in their mid twenties and often married. Similarly, players in American football teams are required to complete four years of college before they can sign with a professional NFL team.

Another trend that undermines the social learning skills of the eighteen year olds coming into top NRL and AFL teams is the abolition of the reserve-grade competition. In the past, quite often a brash teenager on the way up was quietly pulled into line by the wizened 32-year-old prop forward who was on his way down and playing out the final year of his contract in the seconds. St George Illawarra centre Mark Gasnier was fined $50,000 for sending a lurid, sleazy text message to a girl at 3 am, while he was in camp with the NSW State of Origin team; he later moved to France to play with a Parisian rugby union club. Some of the purists in the 'game they play in heaven' initially feared Gasnier would pollute their noble code; later, when his behaviour was seen to be impeccable in France, they gave credit to the superior behavioural standards of 'the gentleman's game'. Rubbish. Gasnier had grown up, taken his French-speaking partner to Paris and had escaped the Sydney fishbowl.

Nor is binge drinking in the AFL and the NRL a reflection of lower IQ. It's a society-wide problem. Many young people, who don't touch alcohol over the working week, leave home at 11 pm on a Friday night to go out and consume heavily over the weekend. Former players are as horrified to learn the modern player can consume twenty beers after a match, just as today's player is shocked to know players of my era drank a few beers the night before a game. In fact, binge drinking in the football codes is increasingly migrating to the off-season, now that players realise alcohol slows down the healing of damaged tissue. If there is a close relationship between heavy drinking and the contact sports, it exists mainly in that window of the year when there is little contact.

In the week of the *Four Corners*' exposure, an American lap dancer, Theresa White, said of her relationship with swimmer Michael Phelps—who won more gold medals in Beijing than any other Olympic athlete in history—'Michael should get another Olympic gold medal for marathon lovemaking. When I ran into another girl called Jen at a party, it turned out he was sleeping with both of us. And I've heard that there are five or six girls he can call on any time to come over and be with him.'

The superstar of Beijing had previously been photographed smoking marijuana at a party. Yet, while Phelps escaped these sleazy sex and drug revelations with his sponsorships intact, the Australian media had turned savagely against rugby league. Okay, the code had some priors but I recall thinking I could never again make the response I once gave when I was asked whether I allowed my players to have sex before a game. That question had been asked during a period when Western Suburbs were being particularly aggressive on the field. 'No, I have no objections', I said. 'Provided they don't enjoy it.' I know I wouldn't get away with saying that now, even with a twinkle in my eye.

To celebrate sport is also to celebrate sheer abandon—it is to savour moments when athletes surrender themselves, hold nothing back and lay it out there for all to see. This is when sport takes all the negative emotions—fear, hate and ego—and transmutes them into great theatre, records, front-page photos and powerful example. Clearly, we love our heroes to be reckless, in the sense of putting their bodies on the line. Of being oblivious to the consequences—whether they're diving for a loose ball on a muddy field, millimetres from prop forwards wearing size 16s; or catching a high ball with their ribs exposed; or being struck by a bouncer. Our sports heroes are people who shoot first and ask questions later.

Off the field, though, we expect them to be the reverse of reckless, pondering the options before they shoot. At one moment, we want them to perform at an other-worldly level and be driven by winning; yet at the next moment, away from the arena, they must behave like we do in our world and not be objectionably competitive. We want to feel that they relate to us—to stop and autograph a shirt, enjoy visiting sick kids in hospital—and yet we hope they realise their good fortune in earning $500,000 for playing a game they love, while we struggle to take our kids to the football once a month. In short, we want them to be both hero and mortal. It is a massive ask but, as I have said earlier, sportspeople sign contracts that commit them to being role models and they must endure it. It's not as if society expects the same behaviour from a greyhound trainer.

The reality is that the personal histories of the athlete and fan rarely connect—the fan never forgets his own great sporting moments, while the athlete rarely remembers his. That long-ago front-on tackle on an opponent stays with some men forever—the rush of air from the rival's lungs, the little groan from the impact and even the snot on his face. We remember forever how good it felt to hit another eighteen year old as hard as we could; yet if you ask a champion footballer to recall something from his playing days, many can't remember anything. I asked rugby league 'Immortal', Graeme Langlands, what he remembered from twenty years at the top and the great fullback said, 'Only one thing. It was when Australia played Great Britain at Wembley for the first time. Davey Bolton made a break and he only had me to beat. If I didn't get him, I reckon the Poms would have gone on with it. He tried to step me but somehow I tackled him and we won the Test.'

There is an awful imbalance in our relationship with athletes, as if we are looking at each other through a one-way mirror. We see them but they really cannot see us. We dress like them, name our children after them and some of us even believe our prayers and superstitions somehow alter their fates on the field. Yet they know only that we are there as a swath of colour in the stands, occasionally as the abusive idiot perched near the tunnel to the dressing room or the pesky fan wanting an autograph. Swimmer Leisel Jones was once interviewed after a big race and shown on a small TV monitor footage of her mother in the stands. Leisel's mother shared the excitement of her daughter's victory with an unidentified male sitting next to her. 'There's Mum with some random,' Leisel observed.

The first sport to understand—even exploit—the great disconnect between athletes and spectators was professional wrestling. In the early days, the wrestlers travelled together. They arrived at their city hotels in the same vehicle but after the event would separate and link up several streets away from the arena so they wouldn't raise the suspicions of fans. They knew fans wanted their wrestling heroes to be heroic and the villians to be evil, the perfect entertainment for the new medium of TV and the moral simplicities of America in the 1950s and Australia in the 1960s. They understood that real life was far more complicated—and ultimately less satisfying—than what masqueraded in the ring as mortal conflict. Killer Kowalski, the American wrestler, knew that his opponent could be a good guy, yet still warrant having his ear bitten off.

They kept their secrets. Who needed to know that Kowalski's great patsy opponent, Bruno Sammartino—whom he seemed to bite regularly, drawing off huge chunks of flesh—was his best mate? For that matter, who needed to know that Kowalski didn't like meat? A strict vegetarian, he bit humans but never swallowed. Akin to President Clinton who admitted to smoking marijuana but not inhaling.

That was then. But today's fans have access to Google, YouTube, Facebook, Twitter, fan sites, statisticians, TV chat shows, newspapers and magazines. They want more and more gossip and information on the personal habits of sportspeople, particularly the sexual. Talkback radio—the modern-day equivalent of gossiping over the back fence—disseminates the information and entrenches the celebrity culture. We want to know our heroes more; but their response is to like us less.

Fans have an ever-expanding arsenal of communication including hand-held video cameras and 'rumour files' on radio through which to convey the latest athlete 'outrage' to the media. The fan who photographs the footballer on his or her mobile phone becomes part of the story and, by extension, famous as well. A 27-year-old supporter of NRL club Cronulla feigned a terminal illness to fraudulently receive a half-million-dollar payout from an insurance company. After sending cheques for $30,000 to the Sharks, he then went on TV to denounce the club's chief executive for hiding the money, thereby guaranteeing his Andy Wahol fifteen minutes of fame. Or its modern equivalent—an entry in Wikipedia.

Newspaper editors, aware the electronic media is like an army charging over the hill, want the latest celebrity story before the opposition pays for it. Competition between and within the types of media is intense. TV's fifteen-second grab must be countered by the tabloid's pithy quote on the back page. Can you believe that 60 years ago, American baseballer Joe DiMaggio, when asked for a quote, mistook it for a soft drink? The hydra-headed monster called the media has grown in tandem with fans' need for information, particularly those titbits that appear on tabloid pages titled 'Confidential'.

Fame and infamy can be delivered instantly by a media who confuse the public's right to know with its need to tell. AFL player Ben Cousins, the redeemed drug addict, was monitored in a manner that made him appear, as one writer said, as if he was Dorian Gray meets Dr Jeckyl and Mr Hyde meets the Prodigal Son. Cousins observed a fixed TV camera in the visitor's dressing room hours before his match; he gave it a single-finger salute, commonly called the 'bird', expecting this to be seen only by the operator in the outside broadcast van. Yet it led the nightly national news broadcast. Who is more culpable? Cousins for doing it, or the televiser for showing it? Cousins was fined by his club and the AFL. Dealing with the media is as requisite a skill as slotting a goal or sinking a putt.

The AFL has clumsily attempted to tap into the vacuous, celebrity-obessed popular culture by re-branding its Brownlow medal presentation night as a red-carpet fashion show for WAGs (wives and girlfriends) attended by some football stars. At the 2009 night, former Sydney Swans owner, Geoffrey Edelsten—a doctor who had spent time in jail for hiring a hitman to assault a former patient—strolled along the carpet with a big-busted woman who according to one observer, looked as if she was simultaneously head-locking two bald men.

The TV cameras also focused on Carlton star Brendan Fevola getting seriously drunk. Fevola was to tape a segment for *The Footy Show* but it was canned after he vomited on the carpet, attempted to assault a TV producer and propositioned a female journalist. Carlton traded Fevola to the Brisbane Lions and the AFL made some comments about his inappropriate behaviour, but then arranged the 2010 draw to accommodate two games between Carlton and Brisbane. AFL officials even admitted the fixture list (should that be simply, fix?) was varied to capitalise on the publicity Fevola generated. The first game, an Easter Thursday 'blockbuster', fell on 1 April and the second on 1 July—April Fools' Day and the start of the new financial year, respectively. Three years earlier, Fevola, despite being married, was involved in an affair with model Lara Bingle. He photographed her on his mobile phone while she was under the shower and the shocked look on her face indicated she did not approve. The relationship eventually ended and Lara took up with Michael Clarke, the vice-captain of the Australian cricket team. They became engaged; moved into an apartment overlooking Bondi Beach and Lara drove a smart sports car or walked her two Pomeranians along the beachfront. It seemed she would live happily ever after until a women's magazine ran off with the 'ever after' and spliced in one of those teary endings you see in Cannes. The magazine printed the shower photos. Lara was horrified and took legal action against Fevola. The AFL, sensing a developing soap opera, announced Fevola had breached its respect and responsibility code and encouraged Lara to contact them. But she did something very stupid . . . she employed a celebrity agent, Max Markson, who sold her side of the story to . . . the same magazine that printed the shower scene.

Clarke was furious. He flew from New Zealand where the Australian team was playing a series against the Kiwis to confront Bingle. Former players railed about him leaving the team, prompting newspapers to run an online poll: 'Should Michael have walked out on his team mates?' He broke off the engagement and talk in the gossip magazines was that Lara had thrown her 4.7 carat diamond engagement ring down the toilet. Michael was later photographed being consoled by a gorgeous Canadian blonde in a Sydney bar.

Each morning during this saga, I checked developments online in the *SMH*. Any doubts about the public's fascination with this blurring of sport and celebrity would be dispelled by the notation beside each day's development: 'You are one of 167 people reading this.' Click to a standard sport story and it's usually five people. Oh, and the AFL finally announced no action would be taken against Fevola. He admitted taking the photo but denied sending it to anyone. The victim and the villain had swapped places. Bingle, photographed without her consent, lost her fiancé and her credibility, while poor Brendan had been cruelly embarrassed by someone sneaking a look at his mobile phone and sending a snap to a women's magazine.

The academics argue sportsmen are society's surrogates, the gladiators for our pathetic, pitiful egos. They claim we have attended down the ages medieval jousts, cock fights, football matches and boxing bouts, to see others act out our aggressions. Even those who hate sport maintain it is healthy for the spectator psychologically because of the collective release of weekly pent-up anger. Yet I've seen crowds become more violent as the play became more physical, and I've seen crowds boo when it got out of hand. Stand on the sideline at a suburban soccer match and listen to the parental abuse; then, as someone suggested, ask yourself the question: if we had more football, would we have less war?

If the atmosphere in modern stadiums sometimes resembles the Colosseum, today's athletes resemble ancient Greeks more than ancient Romans. Songs were written about the Greeks, as they are about today's heroes. No AFL grand final begins without the 100,000 crowd rising to its feet and singing 'Up There Cazaly', an anthem to a South Melbourne player of the 1920s, Roy Cazaly. Ancient Greece's champions were exempted from taxes, while modern heroes enjoy the gifts of grateful governments. Weightlifter Naim Süleymanoğlu enjoyed a flight home to Istanbul in the personal jet of Turkey's president after winning a gold medal in Seoul. Earlier, the Turkish Government had paid Bulgaria a million dollars worth of potatoes in exchange for Naim defecting to Turkey. Most modern nations have publicly funded sports factories and some, such as France, allow liberal tax concessions in the form of 'image rights', where the athlete can receive a tax concession for his picture being published in the media. Image rights as an income deduction are a powerful incentive to overseas stars to play in France.

According to Greek legend, their athletes were immortal. Ours aren't, but they are named so—rugby league originally decreed four Immortals, then added another two, but only one (Souths fullback Clive Churchill) is dead in the biological sense. Married women were not allowed into the ancient Olympics as either spectators or competitors, but single women were the prize. The first prize in the wrestling competition of the games of 546 BC was a woman skilled in handiwork . . . or four oxen. Single women were allowed to attend the ancient Olympics—a veritable meat market of virgins ogling the nude, oiled male athletes and fluttering their eyelashes in search of a husband. Okay, maybe the single women standing outside football dressing rooms today aren't as chaste but . . . you get the idea not much has changed in two-and-a-half millenia.

Or has it? While watching the women's beach volleyball at the 2004 Athens Olympics, it occurred to me maybe the sexes have swapped places. Spectators were seated parallel to the court, while the ends were reserved for the VIPs and the media. The stands were packed with leering Greek men, angry because they were denied the rear view of the bikini-clad beauties who communicate tactics via outstretched fingers on their buttocks—the forward player signals her choice of serve-and-return strategy by spreading combinations of her fingers on her bikini bottom. It drove the predominantly Greek male crowd crazy. They were anxious to sit in the many vacant end zone seats and had a running battle with security who denied them access.

But by and large, spectators today are well-behaved at sporting events, except for soccer hooligans, the occasional streakers and annoying drunks. The 'British disease'—where mounted police herd supporters of opposition soccer clubs into caged areas on different sides of the stadiums—has not spread to Australia, the United States or most of Europe. Advanced technology allows us to be wired to headsets that provide commentary and to watch replays on the big screen, but we still communicate with the man in the next seat. We are a social and gregarious species, forever moved by swirls of banners, the sight of marching bands, the sound of club songs and, yes, the smell of hot dogs. We continue to seek moments when we can connect.

Two memories endure. One followed the best rugby league grand final I have seen: Newcastle versus Manly in 1997—the year the Super League war between two warring billionaires, Rupert Murdoch and Kerry Packer, meant there were two competitions. The code itself was on its knees but the players in the establishment competition rescued it. Newcastle won in the last six seconds with a try engineered by Andrew Johns. A tattooed Maori wearing a Knights jumper high-fived with a Manly supporter who wore an expensive sports jacket and a look on his face which said, 'That's sport'.

The other was perhaps my saddest memory in sport—other than personal losses. It followed the Australia–Iran FIFA World Cup qualifying match at the MCG in November 1997 when two successive goals to the visitors meant a 2–2 draw, Iran winning on away goals and Australia missing the big show in France the following year. It wasn't so much the frustration at the Socceroos' loss of momentum when a serial pest entered the field and cut the goal net after we led 2–0. Nor was it exclusively the stupid comment of then Soccer Australia boss David Hill, who spied me at the press conference and asked, 'What is a rugby league journalist doing here?' I remember replying I was an Australian journalist and felt the despair of many Australians. This gut-wrenching misery was replicated in the thousands of people who circled the MCG long after the match. I recall going to the nearby Hilton Hotel and drinking numerous beers and afterwards, while waiting for a tram, looking down at the citadel of sport in Australia. The circling bands of gutted fans had thinned not a bit.

Modern arenas are also superior places to the old grandstands where we once sat, with their muddy hills and more pillars than Rome. Today's stadiums are the equivalent of the cathedrals of the renaissance: designed by architects seeking to celebrate their art and perpetuate their memory. I walked part of the Great Wall of China with the Australian architect who designed the Water Cube, the arena where the swimmers competed during the Beijing Olympics. Referring to the Cube, he told me softly, 'It's mine'—almost as if it represented his life's work. The Bird's Nest, the adjacent Beijing stadium, used for track and field, is equally impressive and imaginative.

We occasionally gripe at stadium security, at the exorbitant prices for food and drink, at being elbowed out of armrests and kneecapped in seats so shallow you feel as if you have been flying economy class to Helsinki. We moan about the post-game hour-long vanhunt for our vehicle in poorly lit parking areas outside stadiums. We become angry when inflated ticket prices at grand finals mean the seats are taken by corporates who have no emotional capital in the outcome of the contest and make little noise. We shake our head in wonder at the members' section of the stadium when they refuse to join the Mexican Wave, probably for fear their sushi will roll from their plates. We protest they should be subject to surprise interrogations in which they are required to know the score and the names of at least two players per team. They remind us of Bill Veeck, a former owner of the Chicago White Sox baseball team. 'I have discovered in twenty years of moving around a ball park, that knowledge of the game is usually in inverse proportion to the price of the seats,' Veeck once said. But our increasing attendance at events, despite live televised coverage, show that sport really does matter.

Everyone shares a common language now, thanks to sport. It's supplemented the weather in how we communicate with each other—discussions of ethnicity, gender, equity, sex and drugs are likely to take place in the context of sport at the bar or over the water cooler. When tennis player Serena Williams verbally lashed a diminutive line judge at the 2009 US Open, people who wouldn't know a foot fault from a football became excited as her brain explosion was carried around the world by the global media engine. Even the results of the weekend round on the football tipping competition is a conversation starter on Monday mornings.

When Melbourne Storm were punished for salary cap breaches by being put on zero points for the 2010 season, it threw tipping competitions into confusion. Separate tables were run, with the Storm accuring points for wins. One Victorian Government minister suggested the state's premier should award the team a ship as a trophy if it ended the regular season with most wins—'the premier's ship.'

At its most basic level, sport satisfies the urge of men and women to challenge their physical being. Governments know that if sport is performed well enough, it inspires others to activity. Inexorably, despite obscure organisations like the Anti-Football

League loathing the process, sport changes the social and cultural history of a country. It's not the games themselves, or even the players, that are important. It's the harmonising effect of sport upon our society.

Unlike the Catholic and Muslim countries, we are a nation without a single formal religion. Sport is the civil surrogate. It is our national religion because sport, like a faith, can be a morality vessel, a carrier of values—such as charity and sacrifice. Nothing else can bond a people like Australians, who hold so many faiths, including no particular formal faith at all. It follows that a stadium is crucial for a democratic society, even for a benevolent dictatorship, because it's where all classes and types of people come together, to mix and share in a common public space.

Sport has come a long way from the belligerent atmosphere at Twickenham in the post-World War II period when George Orwell was inspired to write, 'It [sport] is war minus the shooting!' Look at the faces of fans today when games are right. The feeling is exhilarating, transporting. It's like sneaking a blanket over your head when you're a child—the troubled world goes away and nothing outside that secret cave seems to matter. It's a feeling as precious as a little boy's dream. Sitting in a stadium at kick-off is perhaps the only time sport is like life because, unlike other forms of entertainment, no-one can be sure how it will all end.

We should never forget we are in the stands because the players are on the field, not the reverse. Elite athletes will still seek to measure their skills against others, even if no-one is watching. Sure, the money we pay for tickets and merchandise and the advertising budgets spent on TV, bestow wonderful lifestyles on the top sportspeople, but they would still play their games without us. Witness Formula 1 driver Lewis Hamilton doing donuts in a $160,000 silver Mercedes outside the Melbourne Grand Prix circuit precinct, in front of a police divvy van. His car was impounded under Victoria's anti-hoon legislation but his burnouts away from the arena clearly show he loves his calling. However, no man is a hero to his valet and TV has become a valet to elite sportspeople, following them everywhere. Hamilton's hooning was captured on videotape and he was forced into a major media culpa shown around the world. This is why we must be alert to the growing gap between the fan and the athlete. Sport and business have intersected in a way that distorts both and has confused the expectations of those on each side of the playing boundary.

The reason the Tiger Woods story was so global was the mammoth gap between the golfer's public image and his private, secret conduct. Many argued Tiger still didn't get it, approving a Nike-produced commercial where his father spoke to him from the grave, and exploiting the publicity. It brought to mind Joseph Welch's response to US senator Joseph McCarthy during the communist hearings of the 1950s: 'Have you no sense of decency, Sir?' Maybe society will eventually hold lower expectations of the role-model responsibilities of elite sportspeople, as it has with sexual mores before marriage. Alternatively, the athletes may eventually accept the higher standards expected of them by society, but right now the fan wants to know the stars more, while the stars like the fan even less. The sports hero unrevealed is dead.

ACKNOWLEDGEMENTS

Richard Walsh, of Allen and Unwin, encouraged me to write this book and then coerced and cajoled me to the finish line. He was pedantic, provocative and patient, but ultimately successful in forcing me to examine my beliefs on a complex range of issues. Thanks also to Jane Palfreyman and Joanne Holliman who negotiated the book to the printer.

I've covered all sports in the media but realised a long time ago that a detailed knowledge of three particular disciplines—cricket, soccer and motor racing—would occupy so much space in my brain, something would have to be thrown out. I have therefore consulted and checked with my colleagues on the ABC's *Offsiders* program—Gideon Haigh, Francis Leach and Gerard Whately—on these three sports and I thank them for their patience. Also, my colleagues at the *Sydney Morning Herald*, particularly Brad Walter who covered for me while I wrote this book and assisted with the data gathering. Thanks also to emertus professor of rugby league, Ron Massey, who read the manuscript and made suggestions that I obediently followed.

The footballers I coached deserve special mention. Their successes brought me to the attention of newspaper editors and that led me to the columns I wrote and, ultimately, this book.

Finally, I wish to thank my wife, Elaine Canty, herself a pioneer in sports broadcasting. She thinks I write wonderfully, but she would say that, wouldn't she?